RATIONAL DIAGNOSIS
AND TREATMENT

Rational Diagnosis and Treatment
Evidence-Based
Clinical Decision-Making

HENRIK R. WULFF MD

Professor of Clinical Theory and Ethics
Department of Medical Philosophy and Clinical Theory
Faculty of Health Sciences, Panum Institute
University of Copenhagen

AND

PETER C. GØTZSCHE MD

Consultant Physician
Director of the Nordic Cochrane Centre
Rigshospitalet
Copenhagen

THIRD EDITION

**Blackwell
Science**

© 1976, 1981, 2000 by
Blackwell Science Ltd
Editorial Offices:
Osney Mead, Oxford OX2 0EL
25 John Street, London WC1N 2BL
23 Ainslie Place, Edinburgh EH3 6AJ
350 Main Street, Malden
  MA 02148 5018, USA
54 University Street, Carlton
  Victoria 3053, Australia
10, rue Casimir Delavigne
  75006 Paris, France

Other Editorial Offices:
Blackwell Wissenschafts-Verlag GmbH
Kurfürstendamm 57
10707 Berlin, Germany

Blackwell Science KK
MG Kodenmacho Building
7–10 Kodenmacho Nihombashi
Chuo-ku, Tokyo 104, Japan

First published 1976
Second edition 1981
Third edition 2000
First Danish edition 1973
Second Danish edition 1981
Third Danish edition 1987
Fourth Danish edition 1997
Also published in Italian, Serbocroatin,
Dutch, Icelandic and Polish.

Set by Jayvee, Trivandrum, India
Printed and bound in Great Britain
at MPG Books Ltd., Bodmin, Cornwall.

The Blackwell Science logo is a
trade mark of Blackwell Science Ltd.,
registered at the United Kingdom
Trade Marks Registry

DISTRIBUTORS

  Marston Book Services Ltd.
  PO Box 269
  Abingdon, Oxon OX14 4YN
  (*Orders*: Tel: 01235 465500
          Fax: 01235 465555)

USA
  Blackwell Science, Inc.
  Commerce Place
  350 Main Street
  Malden, MA 02148 5018
  (*Orders*: Tel: 800 759 6102
          781 388 8250
          Fax: 781 388 8255)

Canada
  Login Brothers Book Company
  324 Saulteaux Crescent
  Winnipeg, Manitoba R3J 3T2
  (*Orders*: Tel: 204 837 2987)

Australia
  Blackwell Science Pty Ltd.
  54 University Street
  Carlton, Victoria 3053
  (*Orders*: Tel: 3 9347 0300
          Fax: 3 9347 5001)

A catalogue record for this title
is available from the British Library

ISBN 0-632-03197-2

Library of Congress
Cataloging-in-publication Data
Wulff, Henrik R.
  Rational diagnosis and treatment : evidence-based
clinical decision-making / Henrik R. Wulff,
Peter C. Gøtzsche.—3rd ed.
      p. ; cm.
  Includes bibliographical references and index.
  ISBN 0-632-03197-2
  1. Clinical medicine—Decision making.
  2. Evidence-based medicine.
  3. Diagnosis—Philosophy.
  4. Therapeutics—Philosophy.
  I. Gøtzsche, Peter C.   II. Title.
  [DNLM: 1. Diagnosis. 2. Evidence-Based
Medicine. 3. Therapeutics. WB 141 W961ra 1999]
R723.5.W85   1999
616.07′5—dc21   99-044463

For further information on
Blackwell Science, visit our website:
www.blackwell-science.com

Contents

Contents

Preface

'The aim of this book is to show that work at the bedside can present just as great an intellectual challenge and yield even more satisfaction than work in the laboratory. Clinical reasoning can be as rigorous and as logical as that in any other academic discipline. True, the information on which decisions are based contains many elements of uncertainty, but measurement of uncertainty can replace personal and intuitive experience so that reasons for a decision become explicit and subject to analysis'. This is a quotation from the foreword by Professor J.E. Lennard-Jones, MD, FRCP to the previous editions of this book which were published in 1976 and 1981.

The book was written to promote the principles of what is now called evidence-based medicine which at that time was slowly gaining ground. Most clinicians still knew little of the methodological details of, for instance, the randomized clinical trial and many were baffled even by those simple statistical expressions, such as P-values and confidence intervals, which found their way to almost every page in the medical journals. Since that time much has changed. What was then new is now well accepted and regarded as something which ought to be taught at every medical school.

A textbook, however, is still needed and, therefore, we decided to publish a new edition of the book. All parts of the book have been rewritten or thoroughly revised, taking into account the developments during the last two decades, but the aim is the same. It presents an analysis of the foundation of the clinician's decisions when he or she faces the individual patient, and although it stresses the importance of stringent scientific thinking it does not ignore the human aspects of clinical work. It emphasizes the importance of clinical research, but the methodological intricacies are viewed from the perspective of the clinician who wishes to make rational diagnostic and therapeutic decisions, not from the point of view of the researcher.

The latest Danish edition of the book is part of the curriculum for medical students at the University of Copenhagen, and we hope that the English edition may be used for undergraduate teaching at other medical schools. We also hope that it will find its place in the continued education of medical practitioners.

Many of the ideas expressed on the pages of this book were developed in close co-operation with colleagues, especially Bjørn Andersen MD, Professor Povl Riis, MD, FRCP (Hon) and Vibeke Binder MD at the gastroenterological departments, Herlev University Hospital, Copenhagen, and with Peter Rossel, MA and Søren Holm, MD, PhD at the Department of Medical Philosophy and Clinical Theory, University of Copenhagen. We have also benefited from our international contacts, including members of the Cochrane Collaboration and some of those colleagues who have translated previous editions to other languages. Marion R. Wulff, MB, BS helped us prepare this English edition.

Henrik R. Wulff
Peter C. Gøtzsche

Introduction

It is at the bedside we commence our labors and at the bedside we terminate them. [Knud Faber [18]]

Medical students work their way through books on anatomy, physiology, microbiology, paediatrics, surgery and many other subjects; they have to read thousands of pages and to assimilate a multitude of facts mostly for one purpose, the practice of medicine.

Somewhere along the road the students must also be taught how to utilize all this theoretical knowledge for making the right diagnostic and therapeutic decisions, and this lesson is learnt on the wards and in the out-patient departments. We talk about clinical medicine, and the word clinical is derived from Greek *kline* = bed.

Theoretical knowledge is important and bedside teaching will always be indispensable, but nevertheless something is missing. We shall try to explain this by a number of examples.

The medical student may be shown a patient with a palpable liver and a serum aminotransferase level above normal, and the importance of these findings is discussed. That is useful, but sometimes the student is not taught to what extent physical findings are subject to inter- and intra-observer variation, how the normal range for a laboratory test is calculated, and what is understood by normality. Therefore, he may not be sufficiently critical when later he evaluates the clinical picture of one of his patients.*

The student may also see a patient with changed bowel habits who had a positive test for faecal occult blood which led to further investigations and a diagnosis of colonic cancer. However, he is rarely taught the difference between nosographic and diagnostic probabilities and therefore he will be unable to discuss in exact terms the value of a diagnostic test. Later on, he may

* Anonymous persons are labelled 'he' in chapters with even numbers' and 'she' in chapters with odd numbers.

subject his patients to unnecessary diagnostic investigations and misinterpret the results.

Further, the student may see a patient with an acute attack of bronchial asthma and he may also observe that the attack quickly subsides when the patient is treated with a β-agonist. That may enhance the student's confidence in drug therapy, but his confidence may be exaggerated, if he has been taught nothing about the fallacies of uncontrolled experience. The asthma attack might have subsided anyway, or the improvement might be the result of the placebo effect. Most of those drugs which are used today will be replaced by others within a few years, and the doctor who has not been schooled in critical thinking may well expose his patients to new, ineffective or even harmful treatments.

These examples show that the teaching of clinical medicine as a master–apprentice relationship has its limitations. The apprentice learns to imitate the decisions of the master but he does not learn to assess the basis for the decisions. In contemporary medicine many clinical decisions have such far-reaching consequences that, apart from bedside experience, medical students and doctors must be well acquainted with the theoretical foundation of clinical decision-making, including what is now called evidence-based medicine.

Clinical decision theory, however, is not a well-defined discipline and, writing this book, we faced the difficulty that clinical reasoning is extremely complex and that the thought processes leading to diagnostic decisions are not well understood. It is also difficult to get a good grasp of the knowledge which does exist since it must be pieced together from articles in journals of epidemiology, biostatistics, medical ethics and other specialized fields, as well as from a number of useful treatises [1–17].

It is also important to realize that clinical medicine belongs both to the natural sciences and the humanities, and in this book we shall distinguish between what we call the scientific and the humanistic aspects of clinical decisions. We shall deal mostly with the scientific aspect when we discuss the decision process, i.e. how the clinician makes his observations in the individual case, interprets the data and then endeavours to act as rationally as possible combining this information and his knowledge of the results of clinical research. But we are very much aware of the fact that the two aspects of clinical medicine are inseparable, and the book also comprises a chapter on the humanistic aspect, i.e. the understanding of the patient as a fellow human being and the analysis of the ethical aspects of the case.

The examples from the history of medicine which are interspersed in the text illustrate that clinical practice, to a much greater extent than is realized by most clinicians, is influenced by the ideas and traditions of previous generations of doctors. The lessons from history may help us to avoid repeating the mistakes of our predecessors. We have sought some primary sources, but most of the information comes second-hand through standard works on medical history.

In some of the chapters we discuss clinical research methods in some detail, but the book has not been written for those who are actively engaged in, for instance, the assessment of new diagnostic and therapeutic methods. We only wish to guide the consumers of medical literature who have to be critical when they consider the practical consequences of the research of others. The busy clinician should remember that some knowledge of research methodology is a great time-saver as it enables the reader of medical journals to skip all those papers where the methods are obviously inadequate.

Critical reading requires some knowledge of biostatistics, but we do not expect the reader to have any prior knowledge of that topic. We only wish to introduce basic statistical reasoning and to show that the statistician's approach to clinical problems is closely linked to common sense and rational decision-making. A survey among Danish doctors revealed that their knowledge of fundamental statistical concepts (including P-values, standard errors and standard deviations) was so limited that they could not be expected to draw the right conclusions from those calculations which are reported in most medical papers. They realized themselves that this was an important problem [29]. We have no reason to believe that the situation is any better in other countries.

Although the book is not intended as a primer for researchers we hope to show on the following pages that there is a great need for clinical research both at hospitals and in general practice. Much of the research done today, also by clinicians, is laboratory-orientated and aims at exploring the causes and mechanisms of disease. Acquisition of that kind of knowledge is indispensable, also from a clinical point of view, as it may lead to the development of new diagnostic and therapeutic methods, but, before they are accepted, these new methods must be assessed critically in practice. Good clinical research can only be carried out by experienced clinicians, and research at the bedside presents as big an intellectual challenge as work in the laboratory.

We shall briefly present the structure of the book. In Chapter 1 the clinical decision process is compared to a computer flow chart. The first step is the collection of information, and the formal characteristics of the different kinds of data are discussed. This discussion continues in Chapter 2 which deals with the reliability and relevance of the clinical data. In Chapter 3 the disease classification, which is indispensable for recording clinical knowledge and experience, will be viewed from a historical, a theoretical and a practical perspective.

The diagnostic decision is discussed in Chapter 4. If the truth of the diagnosis can be established by independent means, it is possible to determine the efficacy of a diagnostic test. In other cases the true diagnosis remains concealed, or the final diagnosis may be almost a matter of opinion.

The diagnosis is only a means to select the best treatment, and the next two chapters deal with the treatment decision. In Chapter 5 we explain what we can learn from previous generations of doctors, and the randomized clinical trial, which is the logical consequence of that lesson, is discussed in some detail in Chapter 6.

In Chapter 7 clinical medicine is viewed as a humanistic discipline, and we consider the ethical aspects of clinical decisions. Chapter 8 deals with research methods and biostatistics and is meant as a guide for readers of medical journals.

We hope that the detailed Index at the end of the book will prove helpful when those who use it for teaching purposes wish to find examples and information about specific topics.

CHAPTER 1

The Foundation of Clinical Decisions

Decision-making is ... something which concerns all of us, both as the makers of the choice and as sufferers of the consequences.
[Lindley [30]]

And what does 'outgrabe' mean? Well, 'outgribing' is something between bellowing and whistling, with a kind of sneeze in the middle: However, you'll hear it done, maybe—down in the wood yonder—and when you've once heard it you'll be quite content ...
[Lewis Carrol in 'Through the Looking-Glass']

A person who feels ill will usually seek medical advice, and the doctor, having listened to her patient's complaints, will make those decisions which to the best of her knowledge will help the patient most. This sequence of events is not new. If a patient at the beginning of the thirteenth century had developed an acute fever, the physician would have prescribed some medicinal herb. White benedicta (blessed thistle) might have been the choice, because this herb was said to possess great healing powers when it was taken on an empty stomach and when Pater Noster and Ave Maria were recited three times [31]. If the incident had taken place 600 years later the doctor might have made a diagnosis of pneumonia using the newly invented stethoscope, and would probably have ordered blood letting, customary dietary measures and blistering (induced by dried, pulverized Spanish fly).

The situation today is just the same, except that the doctor has a choice between many more investigations and treatments, and that the decision may have much greater influence on the course of the disease, and therefore on the future life of the patient. The decision to treat a patient suffering from pneumonia with penicillin may ensure her survival when otherwise she might have died, and the decision not to do a lumbar puncture in a febrile patient may lead to her death from meningitis, although she could have been saved.

The clinical decision process

It is not so simple, however, that all positive decisions are beneficial and that all negative decisions—omissions—are harmful. Many treatments may produce serious unwanted effects and many diagnostic procedures (e.g. liver biopsies and endoscopic examinations) are unpleasant and may cause complications. The clinician must carefully consider the consequences of her actions, both for the individual patient, and, as we shall discuss later, for the health service as a whole.

The clinical decision process is complex, but may be illustrated by a simple flow chart (Fig. 1). When contact between patient and doctor has been established, the data collection begins (Step 1). The doctor interrogates the patient, does a physical examination and asks for appropriate blood tests, X-ray examinations, etc. When the examinations are concluded, the clinician

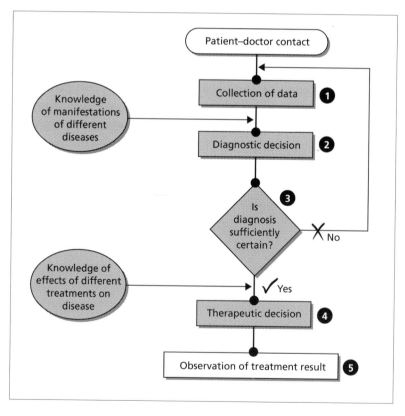

Fig. 1 Flow chart illustrating the clinical decision process.

assesses the data that have been collected and tries to make a diagnosis (Step 2). To do this she uses her *nosographic* knowledge, i.e. her knowledge of the manifestations of different diseases (nosography = disease description, derived from Greek *nosos* = disease).

A diagnosis may be more or less certain, and the clinician has to ask herself whether or not the diagnosis is sufficiently well founded to proceed to treatment (Step 3). If the answer is 'no', the process returns to Step 1 and the investigations continue. If the answer is 'yes' the clinician proceeds to Step 4.

At this point she must once again draw on her nosographic knowledge, this time of the prognosis of the disease and the effect of different treatments. She chooses the treatment which is considered likely to help the patient most, and if the patient progresses as expected, the process comes to an end (Step 5).

This presentation is, of course, greatly simplified and frequently the decisions proceed in a different way. Sometimes the patient does not respond to treatment as expected, and the diagnosis must be revised; and sometimes it is necessary to institute treatment before the final diagnosis is made, as, for instance, in cases of haemorrhagic shock when treatment is started before the site of the bleeding is known. The flow chart also ignores the fact that in chronic diseases clinicians must consider the long-term effects of their treatments, and the presentation does not take into account that doctors concern themselves not only with treatment, but also with prophylaxis.

Therefore, the flow chart in Fig. 1 is by no means universally valid, but it may serve as a framework for a systematic analysis of the decision process.

Clinical reasoning may be *deductive* or *empirical*. Clinicians reason deductively when they base their treatment decisions on deductions from theoretical knowledge of disease mechanisms and the mechanism of action of different drugs, whereas they reason empirically when their decision is based on the experience which has been gained from the treatment of other patients. Imagine that you ask a clinician why she favours omeprazole for the treatment of reflux oesophagitis. Her reasoning is deductive if she argues that the symptoms are caused by acid regurgitation and that omeprazole as a proton pump inhibitor decreases the gastric acid production, whereas it is empirical if she says that usually it has the desired effect (uncontrolled experience) or that randomized clinical trials have shown that it is effective (controlled experience).

Deductive and *empirical* reasoning constitute the scientific component of clinical decision-making (if we use the word scientific in its narrow sense, i.e. 'pertaining to the natural sciences'), but added to this is the humanistic component which comprises reasoning based on an *understanding of the patient* as a fellow human being, and *ethical* reasoning based on ethical norms (see Chapter 7). Thus, clinical decision-making is a synthesis of four types of reasoning.

Clinical data

A house physician at a medical unit reports to a registrar that she has just seen a new patient who presents with a red and swollen left lower leg and tenderness of the calf. The registrar accepts the suggestion that anticoagulant treatment is instituted in order to prevent progression of the surmised deep venous thrombosis. However, another houseman who has also seen the patient objects. It is true that the leg is red and swollen, but the demarcation of the erythema is sharp, the affected skin is raised compared with the adjoining normal skin, and the patient has a small ulceration on the foot. The registrar now correctly diagnoses erysipelas and changes the treatment to penicillin. The example illustrates the well-known danger involved when decisions are made by a doctor who has not examined the patient herself. Both diagnosis and treatment depend on the collected data and no amount of professional knowledge can compensate for incorrect information. Therefore, it is not possible to attempt an analysis of diagnostic and therapeutic decision-making until the information which is used for the decisions has been analysed in detail, but unfortunately this analysis is hampered by the fact that many of the terms which we generally use are vague and ill-defined.

In this book we shall use the term *clinical data* to denote all those data about the individual patient which are relevant for the decision process, and collectively these data are said to constitute the patient's *clinical picture*. Consequently, the clinical data in this wide sense comprise both the data recorded at the bedside (symptoms and signs), i.e. the truly clinical data, and the results of laboratory investigations, i.e. the so-called paraclinical data. Further, the clinical data (and the clinical picture) include negative findings, such as 'the lack of neck stiffness' in a febrile patient.

We shall use the following definitions of the different types of clinical data:

Subjective symptoms. These are the sensations noted by the patient (e.g. pain, clouded vision and dizziness) and the patient's mood (e.g. depression and anxiety).

Objective symptoms. This term signifies all observations made by the patient or the relatives concerning the patient's body and its products, e.g. swollen ankles, blood in the urine or an epileptic attack.

Physical signs. These comprise all those observations which are made by the doctor during the physical examination, e.g. a cardiac murmur, fever or jaundice. Some of the recorded 'signs', such as tenderness, dysaesthesia or loss of central vision of one eye, fall into a special group. They are subjective symptoms which are only noticed by the patient during the physical examination, and they may appropriately be called *provoked symptoms*.

Paraclinical data. These include all laboratory results, and the results of all examinations not done by the clinician herself, such as blood analyses or radiological and histological findings. Paraclinical data may be either *descriptive*, e.g. the shadow on a chest X-ray, or *quantitative*, i.e. the blood glucose concentration.

The patient's record will also contain other data which may be of paramount importance, e.g. information about occupation, family life, previous illnesses, medication, smoking, drinking and other habits.

The erysipelas case illustrated that incomplete or unreliable information may easily lead the decision process astray, and it is worthwhile considering how the clinical data come to the clinician's attention. We may for this purpose distinguish between three types of data:

1   the symptoms which make the patients seek medical advice;
2   the data which are revealed by the routine questioning and the routine investigation of the patient;
3   the data which are the results of diagnostic tests that are carried out to confirm or exclude various diagnostic possibilities.

The first type of data may be labelled the *iatrotropic* symptoms (from Greek *iatros* = doctor and *trope* = turn) [1]. They are the subjective and objective symptoms that make the patient *turn* to her doctor as opposed to the *non-iatrotropic* symptoms which are only disclosed during the taking of the history. In the same way one may distinguish between iatrotropic and non-iatrotropic cases of a disease. A patient who sends for a doctor because of a high temperature and who, during history taking admits having epigastric pain, may represent an iatrotropic case of pneumonia and a non-iatrotropic case of duodenal ulcer. Non-iatrotropic cases may also be diagnosed during a routine medical 'check-up' or at mass screening for some disease.

Iatrotropic symptoms are of particular importance as they usually represent that problem which the doctor, in the eyes of the patient, has to solve, and they ought to be given particular prominence, especially in hospital notes. Nowadays it is not rare in hospital practice that the investigations bring some unexpected findings to light which then lead to further investigations along a side-track. After a while the whole staff is interested in, say, the immunoglobulin pattern, and nobody remembers why the patient was admitted. Only on the day on which the patient is discharged will she say, 'But you have not done anything about my backache!'. The advanced specialization of hospital departments invites the occurrence of such incidents. If a patient presents a complex clinical picture, the subspecialized physician may more or less consciously emphasize those clinical data which pertain to her own field of interest, whereas the remaining data are treated more lightly.

A symptom may become iatrotropic for a number of reasons. One patient with abdominal pain may ask to see her doctor because she is afraid of cancer while somebody else with the same complaint may be worried about losing her job, and in other cases the reason for the visit is not directly related to the symptoms. The patient may have felt a lump in the breast which she dares not mention, but hopes that the doctor will find, or she may have problems at work or at home which made her contact her doctor on the pretext of some mild symptom, which under normal circumstances she would have accepted. Personal problems of any kind may lower the *threshold of iatrotropy*.

The second type of data are recorded routinely from all patients. In hospital practice they comprise answers to standard questions during history taking, the results of the ordinary physical examination and some simple paraclinical tests, such as haemoglobin determination and urine analysis. The routine history taking and examination is to a large extent determined by tradition and from time to time it must be brought up to date. It is no longer necessary in some countries to ask all elderly patients whether they have had rheumatic fever or diphtheria, but it is important to ask detailed questions about their social network and their living conditions. Perhaps the dangers of working with organic solvents would have been detected earlier if the notes contained more routine information about occupation and working conditions.

The third type of data are those collected during the diagnostic process, which begins as soon as the iatrotropic symptoms have been recorded. The clinician will, for instance, ask a jaundiced patient if she has had abdominal pain and or if she has travelled abroad, and such specific questions may well be likened to diagnostic tests, which aim at confirming or excluding different diagnostic possibilities. In other words, the process passes through the loop in the flow chart (Fig. 1) many times during the taking of the history.

Scales of measurement

Clinical data have many characteristics which are not peculiar to medicine, and we shall now consider the classification of data in general terms, using nonmedical examples. A reasonable approach has been suggested by Stevens who describes three levels of measurement [32]: the nominal scale, the ordinal scale and the interval scale.

At a music lesson, a recording of a short passage from an orchestral work is played and the children are asked to identify the solo instrument at a particular moment. Each child is asked to indicate her reply on a list of all the instruments of the orchestra. Such a list, which is used to classify qualitative observations in a series of named categories, is called a *nominal scale*, which from a formal point of view must fulfil three conditions. Firstly, each category or class must be well defined, and we shall see later that this requirement in particular causes great difficulties in clinical medicine. Secondly, the classification must be exclusive, meaning that no observation must belong to more than one category, and thirdly the classification must be exhaustive, which means that all observations to be classified must belong to one of the categories. It is often possible to reduce a nominal scale to fewer classes. In the present example one might have used four classes (strings, woodwind, brass and percussion) or even two classes ('stringed instruments' and 'other instruments'). A scale consisting of only two classes is called a *binary scale*.

Observations may be more refined. In 1806 the British admiral Sir Francis Beaufort constructed a scale for the measurement of wind force. The scale which consists of 13 classes is shown in Table 1. This is an example of an *ordinal scale*, and although it must have formed the basis for important decisions in the course of history it has its limitations. We may take it for granted that a Force 10 is greater than, say, a Force 8, and that a Force 3 is greater than a Force 1, but we must not presuppose that the difference between Force 10 and Force 8 is the same as the difference between Force 3 and Force 1. That was revealed (as shown in Table 1) when it became possible to measure the wind force in m/s. To measure on an ordinal scale is like using an unevenly stretched elastic tape measure, and therefore it makes little sense calculating the 'mean wind-force'. An ordinal scale may also be reduced to a binary scale, which would be the case if we only distinguished between 'windy weather' and 'calm weather'.

The *ranking* of data also provides measurements on an ordinal scale. School children may, for instance, be ranked from the top to the bottom of the form according to their proficiency, but once again one cannot assume that the difference between the proficiency of, say, number 5 and 6, is the same as that between number 6 and 7.

The *interval scale* represents the highest level of measurement. Weighing an object on a balance or the wind force in m/s may serve as examples. In these cases the scale is continuous and the interval, which is constant along the scale, is chosen to suit the precision of the measuring instrument. It may be 1 g for an

Table 1 Beaufort scale of wind force. Specifications for use on land. The numbers in brackets indicate the wind force in m/s.

---

0   *Calm*. Smoke rises vertically (0–0.2)

1   *Light air*. Direction of wind shown by smoke drift, but not by wind wanes (0.3–1.5)

2   *Light breeze*. Wind felt on face; leaves rustle; ordinary wane moved by wind (1.6–3.3)

3   *Gentle breeze*. Leaves and small twists in constant motion; wind extends light flag (3.4–5.4)

4   *Moderate breeze*. Raises dust and loose paper; small branches are moved (5.5–7.9)

5   *Fresh breeze*. Small trees in leaf begin to sway; crested wavelets form on inland waters (8.0–10.7)

6   *Strong breeze*. Large branches in motion; whistling heard in telegraph wires; umbrellas used with difficulty (10.8–13.8)

7   *Moderate gale*. Whole trees in motion; inconvenience felt in walking against wind (13.9–17.1)

8   *Fresh gale*. Breaks twigs off trees; generally impedes progress (17.2–20.7)

9   *Strong gale*. Slight structural damage occurs (chimney pots and slates removed) (20.8–24.4)

10   *Whole gale*. Seldom experienced inland; trees uprooted; considerable structural damage occurs (24.5–28.4)

11   *Storm*. Very rarely experienced; accompanied by widespread damage (28.5–32.6)

12   *Hurricane*. Disastrous results (>32.6)

---

ordinary letter balance and much less for an analytical balance. Interval scales may also be discontinuous (discrete). The number of patients in a ward may be 27 or 28, but not 27.5.

Usually, an interval scale is also a *ratio scale*. For instance, an object weighing 28 g is twice as heavy as an object weighing 14 g. Only measurements on a scale with an arbitrary zero point form an exception. Water having a temperature of 28°C is not twice as warm as water having a temperature of 14°C.

Measurements on an interval scale may be reduced to an ordinal or a binary scale. We may, for instance, measure objects in grams, but for some purposes we may confine ourselves to distinguishing between very heavy, heavy and light objects or just between heavy and light objects. This terminology is useful for the analysis of clinical data.

Taking the history

Often the patient is not able to give a concise account of her complaints and the following example of a conversation between a patient and her doctor may serve as an example.

> Doctor: 'Good morning, Mrs. N.N. What is the trouble?'
>
> Patient. 'I have had an uncomfortable feeling in my chest recently.'
>
> D: 'Have you got a pain?'
>
> P: 'I feel as though I cannot breathe.'
>
> D: 'When does this happen? When you exert yourself or when you are resting?'
>
> P: 'It only happens when I am working; when I do the cleaning I have to keep stopping to get my breath.'
>
> D: 'I remember you live on the second floor; how do you get on going up the stairs?'
>
> P: 'I take it slowly, but I have to wait on each landing'.
>
> D: 'How long has it been troubling you?'
>
> P: 'Ever since Christmas, but it got worse.'

This piece of conversation shows how the questioning progresses. The patient presents a vague complaint, 'an uncomfortable feeling in the chest', and it takes the doctor a couple of questions to be sure that the problem is dyspnoea on exertion. One may imagine that the doctor has in her mind a nominal scale of all possible symptoms, and that she is trying to refer her patient's complaint to one of these named categories. Classification on a nominal scale, however, requires that all categories are well defined, and unfortunately most symptoms do not fulfil this requirement. All doctors may agree that the symptom angina pectoris suggests arteriosclerotic heart disease, but if a group of doctors are asked how they define the symptom, then the replies vary. Some say that it is necessary that the pain only occurs during exertion, others demand that the pain has a typical radiation, and yet others pay particular attention to the effect of nitroglycerine. It always provokes heated discussion when participants in postgraduate medical courses are asked to define common medical terms; there is immediate disagreement with an admixture of aggression as everybody believes that her interpretation is the right one.

The patient in the example had dyspnoea, and that term is also ambiguous as it is used to describe both a subjective symptom (shortness of breath) and a physical sign (visibly laboured respiration). We shall return to the problem of definitions several times in this book, and we shall also point out that it does not matter so much which defining criteria are chosen, as long as there is mutual agreement. Authors of textbooks could do much to bring about such standardization.

It is best always to use neutral medical terms, i.e. terms which do not imply the cause of the complaint, and to avoid expressions such as ulcer dyspepsia, pleural pain, and biliary colics. Such *diagnostic data transformation* is often found in medical notes and it may prejudice the clinician against other diagnostic possibilities. One should not attempt to make a diagnosis until the necessary data have been collected.

When the complaint has been named and classified its degree of severity must be assessed. In the example, the doctor extracted the information that the patient had to stop from time to time while doing her housework and that she must rest on each landing going upstairs. The severity of the symptoms can often be measured on an ordinal scale using expressions like mild, moderate and severe, but first it is necessary to define, as exactly as possible, the individual classes. We may, for instance, talk about mild dyspnoea if it does not limit normal activity, moderate dyspnoea if it limits but does not prevent normal activity, and severe dyspnoea if it prevents normal activity. Such an ordinal scale with predefined classes is often called a *rating scale*, and in the example the patient's dyspnoea is rated as moderate. The severity of other symptoms as, for instance, abdominal pain in gastric ulcer patients may be assessed in exactly the same way: The patient notices the pain but continues working normally, her working capacity is reduced, or she stops working.

In these examples the severity was graded according to an ordinal scale with defined classes, but the severity of the symptoms in a particular patient may also be assessed over time by simple ranking. A patient may say: 'I am feeling better than yesterday, but I am not as well as two days ago'.

A more refined method has been suggested for the measurement of pain intensity in, for instance, rheumatoid arthritis. The patients are asked to mark the degree of their complaint on a so-called *visual analogue scale*, i.e. a line, usually 100 mm long, ranging from 'no pain' to 'pain as bad as it can be' (Fig. 2) [33]. Usually, however, this method cannot be recommended. Everybody knows what it means to suffer no pain, but the other end of the scale is

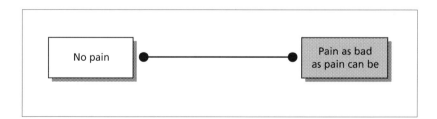

Fig. 2 Visual analogue scale for measuring pain.

left to the patient's imagination, and in practice patients may be reluctant to commit themselves when they are shown the line.

The method also invites meaningless statistical calculations. It is tempting to believe that the visual analogue scale is an interval scale and that it permits measurement of pain in mm, but that is not the case. It is only an ordinal scale, as it cannot be taken for granted that a difference of 10 mm at the lower end of the scale corresponds to the same difference in pain intensity as a difference of 10 mm at the higher end of the scale. Therefore, it makes no sense to calculate, for instance, mean and standard deviation which presuppose an interval scale, and instead one must use ordinal scale statistics (with calculation of median and quantiles) as explained in Chapter 8. It has been shown that the grading of pain in rheumatoid arthritis, using a simple rating scale with four or five classes, is more sensitive than measurements on a visual analogue scale [34].

Finally, the symptom must be assessed chronologically. In the example the patient had suffered dyspnoea 'since Christmas' and this information is recorded as the number of months or weeks, i.e. on an interval scale. In the case of intermittent symptoms the chronological assessment also includes the duration of attacks and the intervals between them.

The physical examination

The physical examination, as it is performed today, originated in France at the beginning of the nineteenth century at which time the so-called Paris School of pathological anatomy was flourishing. Anatomical and clinical observations were correlated, and it became the task of the clinician by means of the physical examination to make those diagnoses which were known from autopsy studies.

Examination of the lungs and heart was developed at that time. Corvisart (1755–1821), Napoleon's physician, made percussion a routine examination and Laënnec (1781–1826) developed auscultation by means of the stethoscope. It is said that once Laënnec had to examine an obese female patient; he could not feel the apex beat and in order not to apply his ear to her chest in an unseemly manner he rolled a sheaf of paper into a cylinder. Auscultation had its golden age before the introduction of radiology, electrocardiography and echography, but it is still of considerable importance. In general practice the decision whether or not to treat a febrile patient with penicillin may depend on the result of the examination of the chest.

Nowadays doctors' expertise in listening to the sounds of the chest has declined, and the terminology which we use to describe our findings is chaotic. Anybody who spends a little time looking up the clinical signs in pneumonia, asthma and bronchitis in different textbooks will be surprised by the plethora of undefined terms. Perhaps we should confine ourselves to talking about coarse bubbling sounds (typically in chronic bronchitis), wheezing (in asthma), fine bubbling sounds (in pneumonia and congestive heart disease), and friction rubs (in pleurisy).

It is possible that computer technology will improve the situation by the introduction of educational programmes where the student sees the examination of the patient on the screen and at the same time hears what the physician hears in her stethoscope. In that way ostensive definitions, i.e. definition by demonstration of typical cases, may replace the usual verbal definitions.

In hospital practice, chest auscultation is part of the routine physical examination, but other clinical examinations are only done on those patients who present certain clinical pictures, e.g. palpation of the temporal artery in patients with pyrexia of unknown origin or examination for ruptured ligaments after a knee trauma. Such examinations represent diagnostic tests which are carried out on the suspicion of a particular diagnosis.

Paraclinical findings

Typically, paraclinical findings are the results of all those tests and observations which are made in the 'paraclinical' departments, i.e. departments of pathology, clinical chemistry, radiology, etc. (but they may also be said to include those simple laboratory tests which are done by the clinicians themselves). They serve a clinical purpose and therefore they are included when in this book we use the term clinical data or talk about the patient's clinical picture.

Radiological, scintigraphic and histological findings are examples of descriptive, paraclinical data. They must, just like symptoms and physical signs, be classified by means of a nominal scale with well-defined classes (e.g. different types of colonic polyps), and they may be graded on an ordinal scale (e.g. slight, moderate or severe dysplasia).

Paraclinical observations are usually considered more objective, and therefore more reliable than those observations which are made at the bedside. This may often be true, but clinicians should be aware of the fact that, for instance, X-ray reports may be biased by the information on the request form, in which case the paraclinical observation may just help to sustain a wrong diagnosis. In order to solve this problem, the suggestion has been made that the paraclinical diagnostician should receive no information about the patient's clinical picture, but that is of course quite unrealistic. A radiologist, for instance, must know which clinical problem she is expected to solve, just as the physician doing a clinical examination will take into account whether the patient is febrile, has abdominal pain or presents other symptoms. However, unnecessary diagnostic data transformation is to be avoided. The radiologist who sees a consolidation in one lung should strive at a neutral description of this finding, and she should not write 'pneumonia' if it is noted on the request form that the patient has a high temperature, but something else if the temperature is normal. The radiologist's expert advice is, of course, needed when the clinician considers various diagnostic possibilities, but ideally the synthesis of the radiological findings and the rest of the information about the patient should take place after the initial description of the films, for instance, at a joint X-ray conference. In clinical research, however, it is essential that the X-ray films are read by a radiologist who has no knowledge of the other components of the clinical picture.

Histological reports present a special problem as the pathoanatomical diagnosis frequently also represents the patient's diagnosis, simply because the disease classification to a large extent is anatomically orientated. It is, however, necessary to be aware of the fact that doctors representing different specialties sometimes attach very different meanings to the same terms. Gastritis is a good example. Clinicians in general have often used, and still tend to use this term as a diagnostic label for patients with upper abdominal dyspepsia who present no endoscopic abnormalities. Gastroenterologists use the term to denote certain endoscopic findings, and pathologists only talk about gastritis if histological sections of a biopsy show inflammatory or atrophic changes.

A different example is provided by the words 'acute' and 'chronic'. To the clinician 'acute' means 'of sudden onset' and 'chronic' is used in the sense 'persistent', whereas to the pathologist 'acute' is synonymous with 'infiltrated with polymorphs' and 'chronic' denotes 'infiltrated with round cells'. A rectal biopsy from a patient with ulcerative colitis usually presents 'acute inflammatory changes' in spite of the fact that the patient may have had the disease for many years.

The concentrations of different substances in the patient's blood are typical examples of quantitative paraclinical data, representing measurements on an interval scale. Such results are usually less ambiguous than the descriptive data, but the clinician should remember that methods of analysis vary and that results from different laboratories may not be comparable.

Global assessments

Up to now we have considered the assessment of the individual components of the clinical picture, but often clinical decisions are based, not only on the presence or absence of a particular symptom or sign, but also on a global assessment of the patient's condition. The general practitioner who visits a child with a high temperature may not be able to make a specific diagnosis and then she will rely on her global evaluation of the child's condition. A child who 'looks ill' may be admitted to hospital at once, whereas the child who seems relatively unaffected will be observed at home.

Global assessments are also essential when clinicians assess the effect of their treatments, both in the daily routine and in clinical research. Therefore, it is unfortunate that many papers in medical journals concerning the effect of cancer chemotherapy only report the effect on survival time. It is, of course, important to know the average number of days which the patients survived when they received different treatments, but this information ought to be supplemented with global assessments of their condition during the course of the disease. It must be reported how they felt, what they were able to do, and how well they tolerated the side-effects of the treatments.

It may be useful for research purposes, but also in daily clinical practice, to formalize such global assessments by calculating a *clinical index* [9] and for that purpose one may use simple rating scales or more complex scoring systems. The rating scales are constructed much like the Beaufort scale (see Table 1). The number of classes may vary, but, if a simple five-point scale is used, one may record at the end of the treatment period whether the patients felt much better, a little better, the same, a little worse or much worse. The ratings may be self-ratings, i.e. the patients' own ratings, or observer ratings, i.e. ratings done by the clinician, but in both cases it is important, as Beaufort did, to define the classes as well as possible. The New York Heart Association (NYHA) classification of the functional capacity of patients with cardiac incompetence is a good example of a rating scale. It uses the following criteria (abbreviated):

1   no limitation of physical activity;
2   comfort at rest, but fatigue, dyspnoea, palpitations, or anginal pain during ordinary physical activity;
3   symptoms even at slight activity;
4   symptoms at rest [35].

In other cases the components of the global assessment cannot be measured on the same scale, and then one must rate each component independently and afterwards calculate a total score. The Apgar score for assessing the state of the newborn is a good example. Here the heart rate, respiratory effort, muscle tone, response to stimuli and colour are rated independently as 0, 1 or 2, and the total score is calculated by simple addition of the five ratings [36]. Other scoring systems, however, are much more complicated. Some anaesthesiologists, for instance, use the APACHE score to assess the prognosis of critically ill patients which includes both a clinical assessment and a large number of laboratory tests (e.g. electrolytes, arterial pH and the white blood cell count) [37].

The calculation of clinical indices may be useful, but it is a condition that they make sense from a clinical point of view, and that is not always the case. More than 70 different methods for assessing the treatment effect in rheumatoid arthritis have been used, and some of them make little sense [38]. In many studies Ritchie's index is calculated. Here the doctor palpates a number of joints, records the pain response on a rating scale from 0 to 3, adds up the results and calculates the total score. In other studies the doctor simply counts the number of tender or swollen joints. When these methods are used, two patients, one with a severe pain in one or two joints and another with a slight pain in a larger number of joints, may receive the same score, although, obviously, the former patient is much more incapacitated than the latter.

Global assessments made by the patients themselves by means of a visual analogue scale are also of little use. The end points of the scale are defined as 'the best imaginable' and the 'worst imaginable' condition which means that their definition is left to the imagination of the patient. In most cases it is better to use simple rating scales with few classes [34].

No matter which method is used, it must be remembered that we are dealing with measurements on an ordinal scale, and, although it is often done, it makes no sense to calculate the mean and the standard deviation (Chapter 8). Complex clinical indices are sometimes referred to as *quality of life* measurements, but this term should not be used in this context (Chapter 7).

CHAPTER 2

The Reliability
and Relevance
of Clinical Data

On the basis of this exercise there were clearly considerable difficulties in achieving agreement between experts. In fact it appeared that if one had involved a fifth interpreter there might well have been no finding on which all observers would have agreed [Higgins, Cochrane & Thomas [39]]

Why did I ask for this pathological investigation? Now that I have the result in my hand, I have no idea why I ordered it. It has, as far as I can see, no possible bearing on the case. Whatever the result, it would not influence the diagnosis or the treatment [Lancet [40]]

The quotations illustrate that we must always consider the reliability of the clinical data which we record, as well as the reason for recording them. This is the topic of the present chapter, but first it is necessary to introduce a suitable terminology.

Imagine a serum sample in which the concentration of the substance 'imaginate' is exactly 80 mmol/L. We send portions of this sample to four different laboratories and ask them to determine the 'imaginate' concentration. Each laboratory performs 10 analyses of their small sample, and the results are shown in Table 2.

In laboratory A practically all the results are correct which means that the *reliability* of the analysis is good. In contrast, the results from laboratories B and C are unreliable, but in two different ways. Those from laboratory B are unreliable as regards their *reproducibility* (also called *precision*), since the measurements vary unpredictably around the true value. They are subject to random variation, but, if we calculate the mean, we get approximately the true value. The results from laboratory C are unreliable with respect to their *accuracy* since they are all too high. They are subject to a systematic error (bias), but they are completely reproducible. The results from laboratory D are unreliable in both respects.

Table 2 Results obtained when a serum sample with a true 'imaginate' content of 80 mmol/L was analysed at four different laboratories A, B, C or D. The mean values are 80, 80, 90 and 88 mmol/L.

Laboratory			
A	B	C	D
80	81	91	78
79	75	90	91
81	85	89	87
80	73	89	95
80	87	91	88
81	80	90	84
80	82	89	79
80	69	90	92
80	78	91	94
79	89	90	89

These terms are useful for discussing the reliability of clinical data measured on an interval scale, but they are also applicable to observations on a binary scale. Imagine, for instance, that several radiologists look at the same X-ray films. If some of them say that the films are normal while others disagree, we must conclude that the reliability is poor. The reproducibility would only have been maximal if they had all agreed, but even that would not have proved that they were right. Perhaps all of them made the same mistake.

We shall now consider in greater detail the reliability of clinical data measured on an interval scale, an ordinal scale and a binary (nominal) scale, but for good reasons we shall not discuss the reliability of subjective symptoms. Patients' statements about their sensations are of course, very important, but obviously it makes little sense to discuss their reproducibility, as it is futile to ask the same questions again and again, and it is also impossible to prove their accuracy, except indirectly, if some objective observation explains the complaints. The observation of a gastric ulcer at endoscopy may, for instance, be said to confirm the sensation of abdominal pain. Nevertheless, one should aim at maximum reliability by defining different symptoms as well as possible and by using a thorough, neutral questioning technique.

Clinical data on an interval scale

Suppose that the biochemist in laboratory B had performed not just 10, but several hundred analyses of the 'imaginate' concentration in the serum sample. These results might be shown in a bar chart (histogram), where each bar represents the number of analyses which give a particular result (Fig. 3a).

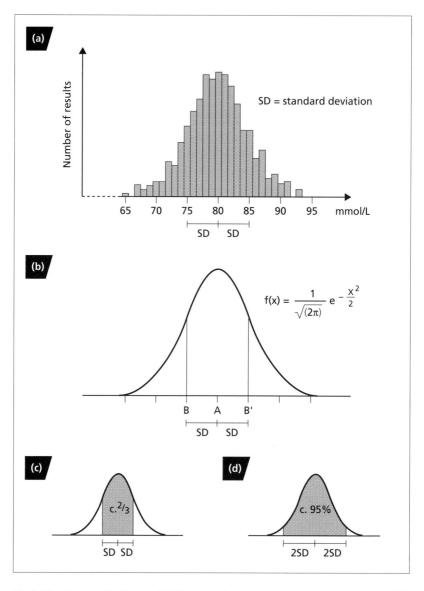

Fig. 3 The Gaussian distribution. (a) Histogram showing the results of repeated analyses of the imaginate content of the same sample. (b) The mathematically defined Gaussian curve (and the formula for the curve, if mean = 0 and standard deviation = 1). (c) Mean ± 1 standard deviation cuts off two-thirds of the area below the Gaussian curve. (d) Mean ± 2 standard deviations cuts off 95% of the area below the Gaussian curve.

It is seen that the histogram has assumed the shape of a bell which, apart from the serration, resembles the curve in Fig. 3(b).

The curve is defined by a mathematical equation, which is also shown in Fig. 3(b), and it is not quite unexpected that the histogram resembles this particular mathematically defined curve. Suppose that the 'imaginate' analysis is very complicated and sensitive. When, for instance, the temperature is a little too high the result of the analysis will also be a little too high, when it is too low the result will be too low; when pH is a little too high the result will be too high, etc. If in this way the analysis is subject to a large number of small errors which either pull the result up or down, then it is to be expected for mathematical reasons (which we need not discuss) that the distribution of the results will be symmetrically bell-shaped, approaching the theoretical curve in Fig. 3(b). Usually, the small errors neutralize one another, which has the effect that we obtain many results near the mean and only few results in the 'tails' of the curve. This mathematically defined distribution was described by Carl Friedrich Gauss (1777–1855) when he was 17 years old and may therefore be called the *Gaussian distribution*.

If the biochemist wanted to publish his results, he might include the bar chart in his paper, but he may also feel that it is sufficient to communicate the mean and the standard deviation. The standard deviation (*s*) is calculated by the following formula:

$$s = \sqrt{\frac{\sum (x-\bar{x})^2}{N-1}}$$

where N is the number of observations, x the individual observations and $\bar{x}$ the mean.

Once again it is not necessary to worry about the mathematics, but let us just assume that the standard deviation, when it is calculated according to this formula, is found to be 5 mmol/L. It is much more important to understand what this result really means, and for that purpose the interval mean ± 1 standard deviation has been marked in Fig. 3(a) and Fig. 3(b). In Fig. 3(a) it reaches from 75 to 85 mmol/L and in Fig. 3(b) from B to B'. We may then draw perpendiculars through these points and it will be seen that they intersect the curve at its points of inflexion, i.e. the points where the curve changes from being convex to being concave. Thus, the mean tells us where the top of the curve is, and the standard deviation tells us where the points of inflection are located.

These considerations are of great practical interest, as it is possible (by means of the equation) to calculate that the area under the curve between the perpendiculars, i.e. the area corresponding to mean ± 1 standard deviation, constitutes approximately two-thirds of the total area (Fig. 3c). Consequently, it must be expected in this case that two-thirds of the results fell within the region 80 ± 5 mmol/L or between 75 and 85 mmol/L. Similarly, it can be calculated that the area corresponding to mean ± 2 standard deviations makes up approximately 95% of the total area. Therefore, approximately 95% of the results of the analyses ranged from 70 to 90 mmol/L (Fig. 3d).

Assuming that the distribution of the results is approximately Gaussian, the standard deviation may be used to indicate the reproducibility of quantitative analyses. Or, alternatively, one may calculate the *variation coefficient*, which is just the standard deviation as a percentage of the mean. This calculation has the advantage that the result is independent of the unit of measurement. In most cases of repeated measurements of the same sample the Gaussian assumption is reasonable, but it is quite possible to imagine an analysis where the errors produce a skew distribution, and then it makes little sense to report the standard deviation.

In this example the analysis was accurate as the mean of all the repeated analyses equalled the true concentration. If that had not been the case, i.e. if the analysis had been subject to a systematic error as in laboratories C and D (Table 2), the difference between the calculated mean concentration and the true concentration could be used to indicate the degree of bias.

Blood pressure measurements are done at the bedside and may therefore be regarded as physical signs, but, since they are recorded on an interval scale, they may also be discussed in this context. If several doctors measure the blood pressure of the same patient, using an ordinary sphygmomanometer, the reproducibility will not be perfect, as they will position the cuff a little differently and as they will not register the change in the sound of the pulse beat at exactly the same time. The results may resemble those in Fig. 3(a), but probably they will also reveal a particular type of bias. It is well known that there is a tendency to record the blood pressure as multiples of 5, for which reason it is more likely that a manometer reading will be, say, 150 or 155 than 152. The accuracy of the readings could be determined by intra-arterial blood pressure measurement.

Measurement of the body temperature illustrates well that the reliability depends on the trial setting. In Denmark, we gave up using rectal mercury thermometers some years ago, and instead we introduced electronic oral thermometers. They gave reproducible and accurate results when they were dipped into warm water, but in practice they proved very unreliable compared with rectal readings [41]. Then, electronic temperature measurement in the ear was introduced, but unfortunately, that does not seem to have solved the problem [42]. The reliability of these methods ought to have been tested in a clinical setting before they were introduced, but that was not done.

The reliability of the 'imaginate' analysis would also depend on the circumstances. It would undoubtedly have been much lower if the laboratory had done the repeated analyses of the sample as part of the daily routine on successive days. Then they would have been carried out by different laboratory technicians, and it might have been necessary to use a succession of batches of the reagents.

Clinical data on an ordinal scale

Measurements on an ordinal scale play a very important role, both in clinical practice and in clinical research. As explained in the preceding chapter, simple rating scales may be used to grade the severity of symptoms and clinical indices to make global assessments, but unfortunately those who introduce such methods do not always make sure that the reproducibility is satisfactory. Often it is found to be very poor.

Usually, the accuracy cannot be assessed, except indirectly if the global assessment serves a diagnostic or prognostic purpose. Then one may correlate the clinical index to the diagnosis or prognosis of the individual patients.

Clinical data on a binary scale

Descriptive paraclinical findings

In the 1950s Yerushalmy and co-workers [43] did a very large study, where 10 doctors read almost 15 000 small chest films taken as part of a screening programme for tuberculosis among college students. They were asked whether the films were positive or negative, a positive film being one which raised the suspicion of pulmonary tuberculosis to such an extent that the reader would like to see a 'large' chest film of the patient. In all, 1307 films were interpreted as 'positive' by one or more observers, and by an elaborate decision process involving a panel of 'expert radiologists' it was decided in the end that in 249 patients the films were 'truly positive' in the sense that these patients required further examination. A further analysis of the results showed that, on average, each reader interpreted 39% of the 'truly positive' films as negative and 1.2% of the 'truly negative' films as positive. The use of the expressions 'truly positive' and 'truly negative' give the impression that Yerushalmy and his co-workers had assessed the accuracy of the readings, but of course that was not the case as nobody can decide the truth of the statement that a patient is in need of further examination to exclude or confirm pulmonary tuberculosis. In fact, only 8 of the 249 students were found to have active tuberculosis, and the study only provides the information that the reproducibility was rather poor, or, using another expression, that the *inter-observer agreement* was low.

Yerushalmy and co-workers have also carried out an *intra-observer study* in which the same observers read the same films twice [44] and this time the reproducibility was somewhat better.

These projects raised a lot of discussion at the time. They inspired further studies which gave similar results and there can be no doubt that the reproducibility of descriptive clinical data is an important issue. The quotation which introduces this chapter refers to a much more recent study where four experienced cardiologists looked at 537 ECGs and were asked to tell whether the ECG pattern raised a suspicion of ischaemic heart disease. One or more cardiologists thought so in 20.3% of the cases, but all four agreed in only 3.7% of the cases [39].

A statistical method, *kappa statistics*, has been developed which permits assessment of the reproducibility, i.e. the inter- or intra-observer agreement, independently of the accuracy [45,46]. We can illustrate this method by means of a simple intra-observer study.

Sixty patients suspected of pulmonary embolism were subjected to pulmonary scintigraphy, and in 22 cases the scintigram was found to be positive [47]. Some months later, the scintigrams were re-read, and this time 14 were

Table 3 Inter-observer variation of pulmonary scintigraphy. (a) Results of dual reading of 60 pulmonary scintigrams. (b) Expected chance results if the diagnoses were mutually independent.

(a)

| | | 2nd Reading | | |
		Positive	Negative	*Total*
1st Reading	Positive	11	11	*22*
	Negative	3	35	*38*
	Total	*14*	*46*	*60*

(b)

| | | 2nd Reading | | |
		Positive	Negative	*Total*
1st Reading	Positive	5.13	16.87	*22.00*
	Negative	8.87	29.13	*38.00*
	Total	*14.00*	*46.00*	*60.00*

interpreted as positive. The results are shown in Table 3(a), which reveals that 11 scintigrams were positive and 35 negative at both readings.

This measure of observer agreement is, however, quite misleading, as it does not take into account that the two readings will sometimes give the same result by chance. Imagine that the observer had not even looked at the scintigrams, but had simply selected some at random which he then said were 'positive'. The first time he had selected 22 scintigrams and the second time 14. Then the frequency of positive findings would be 22/60 and 14/60, and the probability that a scintigram would be labelled positive both times would be 22/60 × 14/60. Consequently, as there were 60 patients, we should expect that 22/60 × 14/60 × 60 scintigrams = 5.13 scintigrams would be labelled positive at both readings simply by chance. Similarly, it would be expected that (38 × 46)/60 = 29.13 scintigrams would be labelled negative both times (as the number of negative scintigrams at the two readings was 38 and 46). These expected results are shown in Table 3b and we may conclude that the expected rate of chance agreement is (5.13 + 29.13)/60 = 0.57 or 57%. When this calculation is taken into account, the observed agreement rate of 77% is less impressive, as it is only 20% higher than the chance agreement.

This approach to the problem has been formalized by the introduction of a statistic called κ (kappa) which relates the level of observed agreement to the level of chance agreement. In this case kappa is 47% as the difference between observed agreement and chance agreement (77%–57%) is only 47% of the difference between perfect agreement and chance agreement (100%–57%). This idea is best explained by marking the agreement rates on a line as shown in Fig. 4. On this line the observed agreement rate (Point C) is situated 70% of the way from total disagreement (Point A) to perfect agreement (Point D), but it is only situated 47% of the way from expected chance agreement (Point B) to perfect agreement (D).

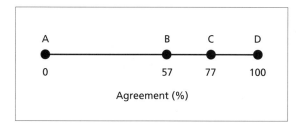

Fig. 4 Calculation of kappa. A: total disagreement. B: expected chance agreement. C: observed agreement. D: perfect agreement. The figures refer to the example shown in Table 3.

The formal definition of κ is:

$$\kappa = \frac{p_o - p_c}{1 - p_c}$$

where p_o is the observed and p_c is the expected chance agreement.

In principle, kappa may vary between -1 and $+1$. Kappa is $+1$ if the agreement is perfect; it is positive (but < 1) if the agreement is less than perfect, but larger than that expected by chance; and it is 0 if the agreement equals expected chance agreement. A negative kappa value makes little sense, as it suggests a systematic disagreement between the observers.

Kappa calculations present statistical problems [48], but are helpful when clinicians wish to assess the reproducibility of the results of diagnostic tests. They provide no information about the accuracy of the test results which must be assessed by means of those methods which are explained in Chapter 4.

The scintigraphy study is an example of an intra-observer study. It would have been an inter-observer study if two observers had assessed the same photos, but the calculations would have been just the same. Many such studies have been done [49], and frequently the agreement is smaller than expected. Gjørup and co-workers, for instance, studied the inter-observer agreement at gastroscopy. The kappa values were 0.59 for the diagnosis of gastric ulcers and 0.54 for the diagnosis of duodenal ulcers [50,51]. These results usually surprise gastroenterologists who believe that their observations are much more reliable.

Descriptive physical signs

The reproducibility of the observations which we make on the daily ward-round is far from perfect, as it is often seen that doctors who examine the same patient disagree. That liver which was felt 3 cm below the costal margin on the Monday may no longer be palpable on the Tuesday, but perhaps a small goitre is found instead which was not demonstrated the day before.

Gjørup and co-workers studied the reproducibility of clinical signs when doctors examine their patients' chests by auscultation and percussion. Each of 202 newly admitted patients in a medical ward [52] was examined by two doctors selected at random from all members of the medical staff. The kappa values, which are shown in Table 4, were far from impressive, considering the fact that the doctors knew that they participated in a scientific study and probably did their best. Before the results were disclosed the doctors were asked to guess what the agreement would be like. This was done indirectly by means of

Table 4 Inter-observer agreement at chest examination (auscultation and percussion). Selected results. The table shows the achieved kappa values and in brackets the expected kappa values.

Rhonchi	0.55	(0.82)
Fine moist sounds	0.36	(0.65)
Coarse moist sounds	0.15	(0.87)
Diminution of breath sounds	0.16	(0.75)
Prolonged expiration	0.53	(0.86)
Dullness	0.34	(0.79)

numerical examples, which permitted the calculation of an 'expected kappa value'. The average 'expected kappa values' are shown in Table 4 in brackets and it is quite clear that the actual results did not fulfil the expectations. In this way the study illustrates that clinicians tend to overestimate the reliability of their observations.

The accuracy of clinical signs can only be assessed if it is possible to determine the truth by some other method. When clinicians inspect the patient's conjunctiva they sometimes state that the patient is anaemic, and when they palpate the abdomen they may make a diagnosis of ascites. In such cases it is possible to assess the accuracy by determining the haemoglobin concentration of the blood or by doing an ultrasound scan of the abdomen, and it has been shown that very often the clinical diagnoses are wrong [53,54]. In general, it is best to avoid diagnostic data transformation altogether, and to record only what was actually observed, e.g. paleness of the conjunctiva or a swollen abdomen (with perhaps absence of liver dullness). These clinical signs may not be reliable for diagnostic purposes, but they are still important as they suggest further investigations.

There are many reasons for the low reproducibility of some descriptive paraclinical and clinical data. Experience and thoroughness are important, but even experienced observers may disagree about definitions, or about the threshold of normality when there is a gradual transition between the normal and the abnormal. In many cases the situation could be improved by better training and by generally recognized definitions, for instance in the form of ostensive definitions (p. 6). The doctors who studied the reliability of pulmonary scintigraphy (as reported above) reached higher agreement when they repeated the study, after having standardized their descriptions.

Further, the examination will be more thorough and the threshold for recording a physical sign as abnormal will be lower if the diagnosis is already expected. We have mentioned earlier that radiologists may be biased by the information on the request form (p. 17), and that a physician doing a physical examination will be influenced by his knowledge of the patient's clinical picture. This risk of bias is inherent in clinical practice, but awareness of the problem may prevent the decision process from going astray.

The statistical concept of normality

The sum of the normal and abnormal clinical data which have been collected by the clinician constitute the patient's clinical picture, and all this information serves a variety of purposes. It may be used to decide whether or not the patient is ill, or it may help to confirm or exclude different diagnoses. It may also be used to assess the severity of the patient's condition, to monitor the course of the disease and to assess the treatment result. But before we discuss the relevance of clinical data for these purposes, it is necessary to consider the concept of normality and the concept of disease.

Doctors discussing their patients often use expressions such as 'the eosinophil count is high', 'the serum potassium is low', or 'the aminotransferase is normal'. These expressions illustrate that clinicians often reduce the scale of measurement from an interval scale to an ordinal scale, confining themselves to a distinction between abnormally low, normal and abnormally high values. They sometimes even use special terms to designate these categories, e.g. hypokalaemia, eosinophilia, hypertension, fever, thrombocytopenia and hypercholesterolaemia. All such expressions presuppose that we know what is normal, and in the case of chemical analyses we usually rely on the list of normal ranges which is issued by the local laboratory. Ideally, these normal ranges comprise 95% of the healthy population, which means that we shall expect every twentieth healthy person to present a value which is either 'abnormally' high or 'abnormally' low.

Imagine a chemical pathologist, who wishes to determine the normal range for a new quantitative blood analysis and records the results in a sample of normal subjects. The distribution of the results can be visualized by a histogram, like the one shown in Fig. 5(f), and, if the sample is sufficiently large, it may be possible to assess the shape of the distribution. It may, for instance, be positively skew (Fig. 5a), negatively skew (Fig. 5b) or bimodal (Fig. 5c). The distribution of the serum bilirubin is positively skew whereas the distribution of the serum concentration of a drug after ingestion of a fixed dose may be bimodal due to a mixture of slow and fast drug metabolizers. No prior assumptions are warranted as regards the shape and mathematical formula of the distribution, and therefore the 95% interval cannot be calculated mathematically. Instead, one must rank all the observations in ascending order and cut off 2.5% of the results from each end. If, for instance, 200 normal persons

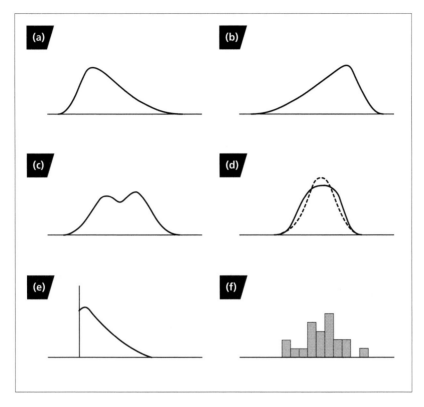

Fig. 5 Different types of distributions. (a) Positively skew. (b) Negatively skew. (c) Bimodal. (d) Bell-shaped but not Gaussian (the stippled curve is a Gaussian distribution). (e) Truncated distribution. (f) Histogram of results from a small number of experiments.

have been examined the lowest five and the highest five results are removed, and the range of the remaining 190 results represents the *observed 95% range*. In statistical terminology the cut-off points are called the 2.5 and the 97.5 percentiles.

Previously, chemical pathologists did not always calculate the normal range in this way. Instead they calculated the standard deviation (p. 23), as they assumed that mean ± two standard deviations might serve as the normal range. This calculation can often be used to assess the reproducibility of an analysis, as there is reason to believe that repeated measurements of the same sample will form a Gaussian distribution, but the Gaussian assumption is unwarranted when we are dealing with single measurements from a large number of individuals. Very often the Gaussian distribution is called 'the normal distribution', but that may lead to misunderstandings, as, normally, biological distributions are non-Gaussian.

Even bell-shaped and symmetric distributions need not be Gaussian as the Gaussian equation (Fig. 3) only fits one particular 'bell-shape', and if we calculate mean ± two standard deviations for the bell-shaped, but non-Gaussian curve in Fig. 5(d), the interval will not correspond to 95% of the area.

Today chemical pathologists are well aware of this problem, but others who report the distribution of some quantitative variable in a group of healthy persons or patients have not yet learnt the lesson. Even the best medical journals publish numerous papers where the authors quote the mean and standard deviation of their results when this calculation is nonsensical. Once, for example, it was stated in a paper that the mean basic gastric acid output in gastric ulcer patients was 1.5 mmol H^+/hour and that the standard deviation was 2.4 mmol H^+/hour [55]. This must give the reader the impression that 95% of the patients produced between −3.3 and +6.3 mmol H^+/hour or, in other words, that some patients produce a base instead of an acid. The truth is, of course, that the distribution is truncated as shown in Fig. 5(e).

This criticism of the standard deviation, however, only concerns its use for descriptive purposes. If the sample is large and the distribution not too skew, it may still be used to calculate the so-called standard error of the mean. The purpose of that calculation will be discussed in Chapter 8.

It is reasonable that clinicians often refer to the normal range, when they decide on the normality of a test result, but they should keep in mind how it was determined. They should remember that it is a 95% range and that, even in healthy subjects, one must expect every twentieth test result to be either too high or too low. If a healthy person is subjected to 20 blood tests (whose results are mutually independent) the probability of one or more abnormal results will be $1 - 0.95^{20} = 0.64$ or 64%. If normality is defined by the normal range, 'a normal person is anyone who has not been sufficiently investigated' [24].

In other cases the relevance of the reference population is questionable. Is it, for instance, reasonable to use a normal range based on blood samples from blood donors or medical students when we decide on the normality of the serum albumin of a 75-year-old woman? Perhaps we ought to calculate a special normal range for the elderly.

The concept of disease

The concepts of normality and abnormality cannot be fully explained by statistical considerations. They are closely related to the concepts of health and disease, as illustrated by the fact that we talk about normal health and as we regard disease as something abnormal. According to the statistical approach, normality is defined as that which is common, and this definition ignores the fact that sometimes disease is common and health rare. Once, for instance, it was normal (common) in Switzerland and some parts of the Balkans to suffer from hypothyroidism due to iodine deficiency, and in many parts of the world today it is normal (common) for children to be malnourished. Therefore, it is necessary to consider definitions of health and disease which do not depend on the statistical concept of normality. This is a central problem in medical philosophy [25], but for the purpose of this book it is sufficient to present very briefly two opposing views.

According to one school of thought, health and disease are regarded as purely biological phenomena. It is taken to be an objective fact that a person is ill, as disease is regarded as a deviation from normal biological functioning, and in this context normal functioning does not mean that which is common, but that which a biological organism needs in order to thrive, reproduce and sustain life. Therefore, a patient with a pyloric stenosis is objectively ill as he cannot thrive biologically unless the passage of food from the stomach into the gut is restored. This biological or objectivist concept of disease may well appeal to scientifically minded doctors, but it is obviously unsatisfactory from the point of view that it ignores that sick people 'feel ill' and suffer unpleasant subjective symptoms.

Therefore, other medical philosophers deny that the concept of disease can be reduced to an objective phenomenon. They adopt a purely subjectivist view of disease and maintain that the primary characteristics of the state of disease are the patient's feelings. This view, however, is also unsatisfactory, as the presence of unpleasant symptoms is not tantamount to being ill. We do not, for instance, say that a woman in labour is ill, but we regard the unconscious person or the person with an asymptomatic lung cancer as seriously ill.

The issue is further complicated by the influence of cultural norms. Once run-away slaves in the western hemisphere were thought to suffer from a special disease called drapetomania (from Greek *drapetes* = fugitive) and Russians who opposed Stalin were regarded as mentally ill and confined to psychiatric institutions. Now we no longer accept these 'diagnoses', just as we no longer regard homosexuality as a disease entity, but instead the 'hyperactivity' of some children and 'the chronic fatigue syndrome' have found their place in the disease classification.

The threshold of iatrotropy also to some extent depends on social norms, and it is possible that some of those people who nowadays seek medical advice because of a mild back pain or an irritable bowel syndrome would previously have seen their recurring symptoms as an expression of the inescapable vicissitudes of life.

The danger of somatization may be mentioned in this context. Personal worries of any kind may lower the threshold of iatrotropy, and the visit to the doctor may lead to somatic diagnoses and, possibly, the institution of treatment. In such cases the net result may well be that the patient's situation has become even more complicated than it was. The personal problems are not brought to light, and the somatic diagnosis causes new worries or even serves to legitimate the role as a patient.

It has become fashionable to propose the adoption of a bio-psycho-social disease concept, which serves to remind us that the disease concept has at least these three dimensions, and that it has proved impossible to define health and disease in simple terms. Clinicians must concern themselves with all aspects of the disease concept, and they must, in particular, take care that they do not pay so much attention to the biological aspect that they forget the others. A few years ago, some well-meaning Danish doctors placed themselves near the cash registers in supermarkets and offered to measure the customers' blood pressure, and those who were found to have an abnormal blood pressure were referred to their general practitioner. These doctors may have done some good as it is possible that they detected some cases of hypertension which, years ahead, would have led to a cerebrovascular accident which was now averted, but the cost must not be overlooked. Some people might simply take it in their stride that from then on they had to take tablets and see their general practitioner at regular intervals, but others would start worrying about their state of health and the effects of the drugs. They would feel that they were 'made ill' that day in the supermarket. Mass screening for non-iatrotropic cases of particular diseases is, of course, sometimes fully justified, but nevertheless this activity contrasts with the classical role of the physician which is to help those people who turn to him for help. It is a different thing altogether to approach people who live their lives believing that they are healthy, and then tell them that their good health is an illusion. It is particularly important to discuss this problem at a time when genetic screening is becoming a realistic possibility.

Regular health 'check-ups' which do not aim at detecting any particular disease are not as popular in Europe as in the United States, and it is doubtful whether they are ever warranted. There is a small chance that a disease responsive to treatment will be detected at an early stage, but there is also considerable risk that the 'check-up' leads to unnecessary worries due to false positive results or to truly abnormal results which one cannot do anything about.

Interpretation and relevance

The development of clinical medicine is best appreciated by looking through old medical records. In the late 1920s the following paraclinical investigations, including routine tests, were carried out at a Danish hospital on a patient who was admitted suffering from severe diarrhoea and anaemia:

> Haemoglobin, colour index, WBC, differential count. Wassermann reaction, benzidine and catalase tests on stools, chest X-ray, barium meal (with follow-through to the colon), and urine microscopy and analysis for proteinuria.

Nowadays a patient admitted for the same reason might easily go through the following programme:

> Blood: ESR, haemoglobin, RBC, WBC, differential count, reticulocyte count, MCV, MCHC. Serum: iron and iron-binding capacity, folic acid, B_{12}, calcium, phosphate, sodium, potassium, chloride, bicarbonate, protein, electrophoresis, creatinine, aminotransferase, alkaline phosphatase, bilirubin, thyroxin. Stools: fat content, test for occult bleeding, pathogenic bacteria, worms, eggs and cysts. Urine: protein, glucose and 5-hydroxyindole acetic acid. X-ray: chest, small gut and colon. The results of these investigations may then lead to others, such as: jejunal biopsy, lactose tolerance test, bone marrow biopsy, pancreatic function tests, culture of duodenal aspirate, coloscopy, serum gastrin and Schilling test.

We do not necessarily imply that any of these investigations are superfluous, but, nevertheless, this example, and numerous others from all spheres of clinical medicine, call for critical thought. We must ask ourselves if the tests that we request are necessary, if we interpret the results correctly, and if they serve the purpose which we expect them to serve.

Probably, some of the tests that we do are not really required. It is customary, for instance, at many hospitals to check routinely the electrolyte status of all newly admitted patients and to measure their blood pressure at regular intervals during the first 24 h. That may often be warranted, but in many cases we do not expect electrolyte disturbances or changes in the blood pressure, and then it might be more appropriate to give the patient the chance of a good rest. Previously, it was also customary to do a routine chest X-ray and an ECG in all medical hospital patients, but in a survey of more than 400 patients with no history of cardiac or pulmonary disease the results did not influence the decision process [56]. According to a Swedish report, many routine investigations before planned operations are also superfluous [57]. In a Dutch trial, where the relevance of the tests requested by general practitioners was assessed every six months, the use of a number of common laboratory tests dropped by 38% over 10 years. In a different geographical area which served as a control the number increased by 52% during the same period [58].

Correct assessment of the results of quantitative laboratory tests requires an understanding of the concepts of reproducibility and normality. Figure 3(a) (p. 22) shows the random variation around the mean when we repeat the measurement of some substance in the same blood sample, and we shall, of course, expect similar variation when we do repeated tests on the same person over a period of time, even when the blood concentration is quite constant. If one day the laboratory returns a particularly high result, we shall, other things being equal, expect a lower result the next day, and vice versa. This phenomenon, which statisticians call *regression towards the mean*, is of considerable clinical interest. If, for instance, one abnormally high result prompts us to institute a particular treatment, we may well be led to believe that the normal result the next day indicates a treatment effect when, in fact, it only reflects the random variation of the results of the analysis. It is better to withhold treatment until we have repeated the test, but even that procedure is not foolproof. We must not, when we see an abnormally high result, repeat the test until the result falls within the normal range, and then conclude that the last result necessarily is the true one.

One must also keep in mind that the normal range only tells us whether or not a particular result is likely to occur in a population of healthy subjects, but that is not the real clinical problem. The clinician wants to know whether the test result is abnormal for that particular patient, and usually it is not possible to answer this question, except perhaps in retrospect. A patient with praecordial pain may have enzyme levels below the upper limit of the normal range, suggesting that he does not suffer from a myocardial infarction, but if the enzyme levels drop to the lower part of the normal range within a few days, it is reasonable to suspect that he had an infarction and that the results on admission were abnormally high in his case.

Indicators

The tests which we do serve different purposes and it might be possible to reduce the number of unnecessary investigations, if we always made it quite clear to ourselves why we request each individual test.

Firstly, clinical data may serve as *diagnostic indicators*, i.e. suggest different diagnostic possibilities. An elevated creatine kinase and certain

ECG-changes are diagnostic indicators of the disease myocardial infarction. The use of clinical data for this purpose will be discussed in Chapter 4.

Secondly, clinical data may be *prognostic indicators*, i.e. serve to predict the course of the disease. The prognosis of colonic cancer is relatively good if the histological examination shows that it is confined to the colonic mucosa, and it is poor if the cancer has spread to the regional lymph nodes. The NYHA, Apgar and APACHE scores (pp. 18–19) are also used to assess the prognosis. Prognostic indicators which are used to predict the development of disease in healthy subjects are often called risk factors.

Sometimes the situation is quite complex as the prognostic indicator may not be the direct cause of the good or bad outcome. It is well known, for instance, that the low mineral content of the bones in patients with osteoporosis predisposes to compression fractures, and, consequently, it was also thought that drugs which induce an increase in the mineral content would have a favourable effect on the prognosis. That, however, is not always true. Treatment with etidronate increases the mineral content and lowers the risk of fractures, but fluoride treatment increases the risk of fractures as well as the mineral content [59]. This example illustrates, what is stressed throughout this book, that theoretical deductions must always be tested empirically.

Thirdly, clinical data are used as *clinical indicators* which means that they are used to assess the severity of the patient's condition at a given moment or to monitor the course of the disease. In everyday clinical practice repeated measurements of the body temperature are used to monitor the course of infectious diseases, and changes in blood pressure and pulse rate provide important information in cases of head trauma.

Patients with chronic diseases who are seen regularly in out-patient departments are, however, often subjected to investigations which are not well suited to monitor the course of the disease. Repeated X-ray examinations of the hands and feet and regular determinations of the erythrocyte sedimentation rate in patients with rheumatoid arthritis are good examples. The X-ray films cannot be used to assess a treatment response as most available treatments have no effect on bone destructions, and the sedimentation rate is badly correlated to the extent of the inflammatory changes in the body. In these patients one may just as well rely on the clinical examination of the joints and the clinical impression of the patient's general condition.

Unnecessary investigations in patients with chronic diseases may even make matters worse. Patients with liver metastases and symptom-free HIV-positive persons should be given the chance to live their lives as normally as possible, and repeated ultrasound scans or helper cell counts may enhance their awareness of the disease.

In general, clinicians pay greater attention to the results of paraclinical tests than to their own observations. The paraclinical results may be more objective and precise, especially if they represent interval scale measurements, but what is gained in reliability is easily lost in relevance. These considerations are equally important for clinical research, especially for the planning of randomized clinical trials. We shall resume this discussion in Chapter 6.

CHAPTER 3

The Disease Classification

'I seem to have an inflamed tongue, doctor. Will you have a look at it?'
'Ah, yes. You have got glossitis.'
'Thank you doctor. It's all right now I know what it is.'
[Conversation quoted by Asher [60]]

According to an old dictum 'there are no diseases, only sick people', and it is indisputably true that no two people with the same disease are exactly alike. Nonetheless, the disease classification is an indispensable tool in everyday clinical practice. The clinician who attempts to assess the patient's prognosis without treatment and with different forms of treatment makes use of the knowledge and experience which other clinicians before her have gained from the treatment of their patients. That knowledge and experience cannot, of course, be transmitted from one generation of doctors to the next in the form of millions of case histories, but only as the collective experience with groups or classes of patients who resemble each other as regards disease mechanisms and clinical pictures. The disease classification represents such a classification of patients where each disease entity functions as a carrier of clinical knowledge.

This way of thinking is also well illustrated by the clinical decision process as it was sketched in Fig. 1 on p. 6. The clinician records the clinical picture of her patient, then she makes a diagnosis, which means that she finds out to which class of patients her patient belongs, and, finally, she exploits the collective experience which has been gained by treating such patients in order to choose the best treatment for her particular patient.

In this way the disease classification may be regarded as a nominal scale with a large number of classes, but unfortunately it is not that simple. Ideally, a nominal scale is exhaustive and exclusive, but the disease classification fulfils neither of these conditions. The contemporary classification which constitutes the backbone of any textbook of clinical medicine reflects the different ways of thinking of successive generations of medical doctors, and it is not logically satisfactory. Sometimes we see patients who cannot be referred to a recognized disease entity and sometimes a patient can be referred to several disease entities. The same patient may, for instance, be said to suffer from chronic pancreatitis or from diabetes mellitus.

The historical perspective

A brief historical account of the development of the disease classification and the changing patterns of medical thinking [18,19,61,62] will make it easier to understand some of the complexities of clinical reasoning today.

The 17th and 18th centuries

In the seventeenth century, university teaching of medicine consisted of lectures, held in Latin, on Galenic, iatrochemical or some other dogmatic medical theory. However, the empiricist approach to science with its emphasis on observation and experimentation gradually gained ground. Thomas Sydenham (1624–84) is rightly regarded as one of the pioneers. He was a friend of the empiricist philosopher (and physician) John Locke and set out to describe, as objectively as possible, the clinical picture and the natural history of a number of diseases.

The following description of an attack of gout which is quoted from the English translation [63] of his *Tractatus de podagra et hydrope* from 1683 shows his abilities as a writer:

> 'The victim goes to bed and sleeps in good health. About two o'clock in the morning he is awakened by a severe pain in the great toe: more rarely in the heel, ankle or instep. This pain is like that of a dislocation, and yet the parts feel as if cold water were poured over them. Then follows chills and shivers and a little fever. The pain, which was at first moderate, becomes more intense . . . Now it is a violent stretching and tearing of the ligaments—now it is a gnawing pain and now a pressure and tightening. So exquisite and lively meanwhile is the feeling of the part affected, that it cannot bear the weight of the bedclothes . . . the night is passed in torture, sleeplessness, turning of the part affected, and perpetual change of posture'.

This description is perhaps particularly vivid as Sydenham himself suffered from gout. Sydenham was the first to distinguish between scarlet fever and measles and he also succeeded in making a distinction between chorea minor and hysteria. He studied a number of the common epidemic diseases of his time, including the Great Plague which swept London in 1665 and in which 69 000 people died.

The need for careful observations became more widely accepted in the eighteenth century. At that time the sum of knowledge in the natural sciences was so limited that many scientists were still polymaths. Botanical taxonomy was *en vogue* and, as many botanists were also physicians, attempts were made to classify diseases like plants. François Boissier de Sauvages in Montpellier (1706–67) wrote *Nosologia methodica* which subdivides 'diseases' into 10 classes, 295 genera and 2400 species, and the greatest of botanical taxonomists, Carolus Linnæus (1707–78) composed a *Genera morborum*.

These early phases of the development of the disease classification are not only of historical interest. The careful descriptions of different diseases which we find in our textbooks follow the tradition from the time of Sydenham and the taxonomists, and we still use symptom diagnoses and establish clinical syndromes, if we have little knowledge of the causes and mechanisms of the disease entity in question.

The empiricist approach, however, did not displace the old ways of thinking. As late as the first half of the nineteenth century many physicians still accepted the ancient doctrines of humoral pathology, according to which disease represents an imbalance of the four humours (yellow and black bile, blood and phlegm), and other equally speculative systems of thought also reached considerable popularity. William Cullen (1712–90) believed that life is a function of nervous energy and that diseases are mainly nervous disorders. Gout, for instance, was classified as a neurosis. Clinicians may still, unconsciously, be harking back to Cullen when they refer to a disease of unknown aetiology as 'probably nervous' [19].

All the speculative theories from those days may be labelled pre- or pseudoscientific, as no attempt was made to test them empirically, but pseudoscientific thinking is by no means a thing of the past. The theoretical basis of homoeopathy, reflexology and other forms of so-called alternative medicine are as speculative and empirically ill-founded as Greek humoral pathology (see Chapter 5, pp. 112–16).

The 19th and 20th centuries

At the beginning of the nineteenth century a new epoch in medical science was inaugurated. Xavier Bichat (1771–1802) published his *Anatomie générale* and during the following decades the French anatomists systematically described the anatomical lesions which they observed on the autopsy table. However, as illustrated by the work carried out by René Laënnec (1781–1826), their studies always served a clinical purpose. Laënnec was both a pathologist and a physician and as mentioned previously he introduced chest auscultation and correlated the auscultatory signs to anatomical lesions found at autopsy. He was particularly interested in tuberculosis and was the first to regard this disease as an entity. It had previously been split up in a number of 'diseases' according to the varied clinical manifestations. The ideas of the French anatomists spread to other centres, including Dublin (Graves, Stokes, Cheyne, Adams and Corrigan) and Guy's Hospital, London (Addison, Bright and Hodgkin). All these names are still remembered as eponyms.

This period of the history of medicine has left its stamp on our disease classification as the majority of diseases are still named after anatomical lesions. We are now so familiar with the tradition that was established in the early nineteenth century that it is difficult for us to appreciate to which extent it represented a radically new way of thinking. The taxonomists of the previous century had not distinguished between the patient's disease and the patient's clinical picture, but from the time of the French anatomists diseases were regarded as something localized inside the body. Physicians, of course, still paid attention to their patients' subjective symptoms, but from then on they saw it as their task to explain the symptoms by the demonstration of an anatomical lesion, i.e. an objective, abnormal finding. Objectivity became the hallmark of scientific medicine.

From the middle of the century it was no longer considered sufficient to describe the clinical and anatomical manifestations of disease. Physicians began to take an interest in the functions of the human organism. Rudolf Virchow (1821–1902), the founder of cellular pathology, gave pathological anatomy a dynamic dimension; he studied tumour growth, explained thromboembolism and was the first to observe leucocytosis. At that time a number of physiological journals were started in Germany and France, and Claude Bernard (1813–78) made great advances in physiology by means of carefully planned animal experiments. He showed in the 1850s that the liver contains glycogen and that pancreatic juice decomposes fat, starch and protein. He also studied the vasomotor mechanism and isolated vasodilator and vasoconstrictor nerves. The interest in experimental physiology led to the establishment of hospital laboratories, where clinicians could carry out paraclinical investigations on their patients and where they could do experimental research. This development has continued to our time and it has led to further specialization and the establishment of disciplines such as endocrinology and immunology. It has also left its stamp on the disease classification. Hypertension, renal failure, diabetes mellitus and thyrotoxicosis are but a few examples of conditions which today are defined in terms of a physiological or a metabolic dysfunction.

The introduction of laboratory research also led to the verification of the germ theory and the development of bacteriology, the pioneers being Louis Pasteur (1822–95) and Robert Koch (1843–1910). A variety of bacteria were discovered, and it became possible to classify diseases according to the infective agent. Typhoid fever, tuberculosis, malaria and measles are examples of diseases which today are defined by their bacterial, parasitic or viral aetiology. The development of microbiology also cemented the concept of 'one cause—one disease' which, among others, even Sydenham had advocated.

During the second half of the twentieth century we have seen the development of molecular biology as a very important new discipline. The molecules in question are primarily DNA and RNA and the demonstration of changes in the genome will undoubtedly leave its imprint on the disease classification in the years to come. It has been established already that many congenital diseases (often rare metabolic diseases) are caused by changes in a single gene, but numerous other diseases seem to be associated with mutations in several genes.

From a philosophical point of view this presentation reflects what has been called the nominalistic concept of disease [25,64], according to which the disease name denotes a class of patients who have something in common, e.g. an anatomical lesion or a functional disturbance. That is what is meant by the expression 'There are no diseases, only sick people'.

The justification of this point of view may seem self-evident, but nonetheless we often talk about diseases as if we accepted the essentialistic concept of disease, i.e. as if diseases had an independent existence. We say that diseases attack people and we describe their clinical manifestations almost as if they were demons, but we must regard such expressions as mere figures of speech. They must not make us forget that the disease classification is no more than a tool which reflects successive traditions of medical thinking. We gradually gain more knowledge about the causes and mechanisms of disease, and consequently the disease classification must from time to time be revised and refined.

Chapter 3

The theoretical perspective

The mechanical model of disease

Modern medical thinking originated in the nineteenth century, and as described above the focus of attention changed from one period to the next. First, our predecessors only saw the structural changes (anatomical lesions) in the body and later on they paid more attention to functional (physiological or metabolic) disturbances, but basically their way of thinking did not change. The fruitful idea which gained ground almost two hundred years ago was the so-called mechanical model of disease, according to which man is seen as a complex 'machine' and disease as a fault in the machinery.

Of course, our predecessors did not overlook the importance of environmental or hereditary factors as determinants of disease. Since prehistoric times it has been known that poisonous berries may cause illness and it was understood, even prior to the discovery of bacteria, that disease may be passed from one person to another. It was also well known that some diseases, such as haemophilia, might run in families. According to the traditional mechanical model, the aetiological (environmental or hereditary) factors elicit the disease process which causes the fault in the machine.

Even today much medical thinking, both at the bedside and in the research laboratory, accords well with this interpretation of the mechanical model. Often, however, it is too simple, and then it may be more appropriate to regard the human organism as a self-regulating system. The organism seeks, much like a thermostat, to keep the body temperature at a constant level, by transpiration when it begins to rise and by shivering when it threatens to fall; it also tends to maintain the concentration of different hormones within narrow limits, and to regulate the blood pressure. Almost all physiological mechanisms are characterized by complex feedback mechanisms which aim at maintaining the normal balance or homoeostasis. All this is well known, but it is worth noticing that this way of thinking leads to a more refined concept of disease. Now the state of disease is not just seen as the end-result of a causal chain but as an abnormal equilibrium of a self-regulating system. The normal equilibrium is health, disease develops when the equilibrium is disturbed, and the self-regulation of the system has the effect that in most cases the normal balance is re-established, i.e. the patient is cured, without medical intervention. This way of thinking may be regarded as an extension of the traditional mechanical model, but it has ancient roots. According to humoral pathology disease is regarded as an imbalance of the four humours and the adherents of that theory saw it as their aim to restore the normal equilibrium by supporting what they called the healing power of nature (*vis medicatrix naturae*). Their theory was false, but fundamentally their way of thinking is not outmoded.

A possible renaissance of biological thinking

The mechanical model of disease, however, has its limitations, as it does not take into account that the human organism is not just an extremely complex 'physico-chemical machine', but a 'living machine'. The mechanical model focuses on the normal or abnormal function of a 'machine' which already exists, but ignores the fact that the human 'machine' is a biological organism which begins its existence as a zygote, grows to its adult form, 're-recreates' itself throughout life, until it begins to degenerate and finally dies. Disease may arise if any of these complex processes run astray.

It was molecular biology which opened the door to an understanding of these processes. We now know that special patterns of nucleotide sequences in the genome may cause serious congenital diseases or just predispose to the development of particular diseases later in life. But molecular biology may also help us to understand so-called acquired diseases. The mechanical models take the 'machine' for granted, and therefore it is not surprising that, until recently, medical science made little headway in its attempts to explain the development of malignant diseases and the degenerative diseases of old age. The cells of our body die and are replaced by others at short intervals, and these diseases are associated with the process of re-creation that takes place throughout life. Colonic cancer is explained by successive mutations in the cells of the gut, and the ageing process of all parts of the body may be seen as the successive slightly deficient replication of many kinds of cells. Anybody who reads medical journals will have noticed the explosive growth of papers on the mechanisms involved, but in most areas our knowledge is still superficial and limited.

In the years to come molecular biology will undoubtedly result in a much better understanding of disease processes, but it is possible that the break with traditional thinking will be much deeper. In this chapter we have used the term 'the mechanical model' which may sound rather simplistic, but from a philosophical point of view it is justified. Scientific thinking in general, including, for instance, physiological thinking, has been 'mechanical' in the sense that it is founded in the Newtonian picture of the world, i.e. a world governed by simple laws of nature. However, during the last few decades we have witnessed the development of new revolutionary ideas which may completely change our view of nature. Different terms are used, and, depending on the approach, one may talk about complexity theory, nonlinear dynamics, chaos theory, fractal theory or the theory of open self-organizing systems [65–68]. These new ideas may help us to understand the creativity and increasing complexity of living nature which Newtonian science was unable to explain.

It is impossible to predict the future development, but it is inevitable that this new world view will have a profound influence on medical thinking and our understanding of disease processes. We shall just give a few examples.

Morphogenesis is still one of the big mysteries of biology. We know that DNA governs protein synthesis, but the mechanisms leading to the formation of the extremely complex structural configuration of a human organism are still largely unknown. Biologists, however, have had some success analysing the so-called nonlinear dynamic processes which are involved in the formation of complicated structures, and they have also shown the importance of environmental factors [69]. The studies were done on algae, but they illustrate the type of reasoning which may be needed to explain the development of disease during the growth phase of the human organism. Studies in humans have shown that under-nutrition of the growing fetus may have permanent effects on body structure, physiology and metabolism and that these effects may dispose to common diseases (e.g. chronic heart disease, hypertension and diabetes) late in life [70].

Fractal geometry also seems to play an important role in human morphogenesis [71,72]. A pattern is said to be fractal, if it repeats itself on a smaller and smaller scale, a property known as self-similarity, and the finer and finer branches of arteries, bronchi and glandular ducts, for instance, may be regarded as fractal-like structures. Such phenomena cannot be explained within the traditional framework of thinking.

In classical mechanics (linear dynamics) it is assumed that small changes of the initial values will only have small effects on the results. This, however, is not so when we are dealing with nonlinear physiological processes associated with complex feedback mechanisms where gradual small changes in the initial values may have striking and unanticipated effects. In studies of isolated muscle strips it was found, for instance, that a gradual increase in the intracellular calcium concentration provoked a regular series of sudden changes in the cardiac rhythm (bigeminal contractions, more complex dysrhythmias and at last chaos, i.e. seemingly unpredictable oscillations) [73]. The dynamics of many such processes have been well analysed, and anybody who has seen a patient suddenly develop a life-threatening ventricular fibrillation will acknowledge that further theoretical studies of this kind may have considerable clinical implications.

Chaos theory may also contribute to our understanding of physiological processes in areas such as endocrinology, neurophysiology and renal physiology [74,75]. Under normal conditions many physiological systems show chaotic oscillations (rather than steady states), and Goldberger has suggested that often chaos is a sign of health whereas disease is characterized by the abrupt onset of regular oscillations [72,76].

Disease and the environment

Not so long ago, on a biological time scale, man lived as a hunter–gatherer. He was from an evolutionary point of view adapted to those living conditions, and since then he has not changed much genetically. His way of living has, however, undergone repeated radical changes and it is not surprising that new living conditions are associated with new diseases. Therefore, the development of disease may also be viewed from the perspective of evolutionary biology [77], and often it may be regarded as maladaptation in the environment.

According to McKeown [78] the population density in the stone age was so small that diseases such as smallpox, measles and whooping cough could not have existed. They appeared by adaptation of animal pathogens when people in larger numbers moved together and established the first agricultural societies about 10 000 years ago. Later civilizations were associated with other diseases, and although it is difficult for us to 'diagnose' the diseases which are described by physicians in ancient Greece and Rome and during the Middle Ages, there can be no doubt that the diseases which they saw differed from the ones which we see today. Now we see the spreading of the so-called diseases of civilization, such as atherosclerosis, diabetes and hypertension to the developing world, where at the same time people suffer from infectious diseases unknown in more developed countries.

The variability of the disease pattern, even during a limited time span, is well illustrated by the history of peptic ulcer disease, i.e. gastric and duodenal ulcers in Northern Europe. In 1881, With, who was Professor of Clinical Medicine at The University Hospital of Copenhagen, published a now largely forgotten book on gastric ulcers [79] in which he related a series of dramatic case histories. Most of the patients were young women aged 20–30 years who were admitted with haematemesis or perforation and peritonitis. Most of them died and the autopsy revealed a gastric ulcer. X-ray examination was not yet available, and therefore the diagnosis could only be made with certainty at the autopsy table. With, however, believed that the disease was common, because cardialgia 'is so widespread in the Nordic countries that few women aged 15–30 years, especially from the working classes, are spared . . .'. According to With, cardialgia was a strong pain in the upper abdomen which often induced the patients to bend forward pressing the abdomen against the edge of a table or the back of a chair. During a period of four years, 339 such patients were admitted to his unit. 85% were women, one third presented with haematemesis, and they constituted about 10% of all admissions. Only one patient was found to have a duodenal ulcer and since autopsies at that time were thorough, it may be assumed that duodenal ulcers were rare. A number of those patients who were admitted and died had previously received the diagnosis of 'nervous cardialgia', 'hysteria' or 'mother-sickness' because the disease often hit young girls who had left home to go into domestic service. Also in those days doctors made the imputation of a nervous origin of the symptoms when they did not know what was wrong. Numerous similar cases were observed in Great Britain during the latter half of the last century. Jennings [80] writes that country practitioners found perforated ulcers in young women, which 'swept away beautiful young creatures within a few hours', one of the most tragic experiences of their lives.

Towards the end of the nineteenth century this disease of young women disappeared and no present-day clinician has ever seen the clinical pictures described by With and Jennings. Gastric ulcer disease is still seen, but now the disease occurs later in life in both men and women.

Then, at the beginning of the twentieth century, the presentation of 'peptic ulcer disease' took a new unexpected turn. As something quite new, numerous cases of duodenal ulcers were reported among young men. That clinical picture is still known, but it has changed throughout the century. Gradually, the patients' age at the onset of the disease has increased, and now duodenal ulcers are seen in both men and women.

We still do not know the environmental factors which caused the gastric ulcers in young women in the nineteenth century, but we know something about the aetiology of duodenal ulcer disease. It seems that the presence of *Helicobacter pylori* in the gastric mucosa is a necessary causal factor, and one must assume that this infection first appeared at the beginning of the nineteenth century. The prevalence of *Helicobacter* infection, which seems to be life-long, has decreased throughout the century and today it is rare among younger people. We still do not know why so many young men were suddenly infected almost a hundred years ago and we do not know why it is not happening any longer. Now we can cure the disease with suitable antibiotic therapy, but probably duodenal ulcer disease would have disappeared spontaneously, even if the medical profession had never found the bacillus. It is a disease of the twentieth century.

The changing history of peptic ulcer disease is just one example of the dependence of the disease pattern on our living conditions. It should remind us that the post-industrial era will be accompanied by new, radical changes in our way of living, and that these changes are bound to lead to new infectious and noninfectious diseases. AIDS came as a big surprise not so many years ago, but our ever-changing environment will undoubtedly lead to other equally unexpected serious health problems in the years to come.

The practical perspective

The disease classification serves to organize all that knowledge and experience which has been assembled by studying individual patients, and that knowledge is then transmitted in a concise form through the publication of textbooks, e.g. textbooks of internal medicine. The books are written within the traditions described above, and usually each disease has its own chapter, the heading of which is the disease name. The structure of the chapters may vary, but typically the information is organized as follows: definition, causes (aetiology and pathogenesis), clinical picture, prognosis, diagnosis and treatment.

Name of disease

Sometimes the name of the disease tells us which patients are described in that particular chapter, i.e. how the disease is defined. It is, for instance, obvious that a chapter entitled myocardial infarction deals with patients characterized by that particular anatomical lesion. But in many other cases it is difficult to interpret the disease name, or the name may refer to an obsolete definition of the disease.

The etymology of disease names provides interesting information about the history of medical thinking. Diabetes mellitus, for instance (from Greek 'passing through' and Latin 'honey-sweet') should remind us of the days when doctors tasted their patients' urine and distinguished between cases where the taste was sweet and those where it was 'insipid'. The disease name malaria reminds us that it was once thought that this type of fever was caused by *mal aria*, i.e. bad air, and in rheumatism with its varying symptomatology it was imagined that the causative agent flowed through the body (Greek *rheos* = flow or stream).

Chapter 3

Definition

The disease name may be informative or of cultural interest, but usually it does not provide a satisfactory definition. As described above the disease classification was created by generations of physicians belonging to different traditions, and textbook authors ought to define exactly which class of patients is described in each chapter. In other words, they ought to fix a set of criteria which are fulfilled by all patients who are said to have the disease and which are not fulfilled by those who are said not to have the disease.

Usually, however, this is not done. Often textbook authors provide no definition at all, or they include what they call a 'definition', which on closer inspection is only an ultra-short description. This deficiency would be of little practical significance, if there was consensus among doctors when they make different diagnoses, but unfortunately this is not so, as illustrated by a classical example from psychiatry. American and British doctors often disagreed how to treat schizophrenia, as the Americans, in contrast to their British colleagues, found that psychotherapy was beneficial. This puzzle was solved when it was revealed that patients, who in Europe were said to have a neurosis, across the Atlantic were diagnosed as suffering from schizophrenia [81]. Somatic medicine offers similar examples. One might think that it would be easy to distinguish between gastric and duodenal ulcers, but there has been little agreement among gastroenterologists. Ulcers in the pyloric canal may be referred to either class, and some gastroenterologists have even held that all those ulcers which are located in the (ill-defined) prepyloric region of the stomach are 'really' duodenal ulcers.

The dearth of explicit, logically satisfactory definitions in the textbooks may have considerable practical consequences. The disease classification serves to organize clinical knowledge and experience, and a clinician cannot utilize the experience which another clinician has acquired treating patients with schizophrenia, duodenal ulcers, Crohn's disease, systemic lupus or numerous other diseases, if they do not use these diagnostic terms in the same way.

It is not easy, however, to define a disease entity. The problems are closely linked to the complexity of the disease classification, and it is necessary to distinguish between: symptom diagnoses, clinical syndromes, anatomically defined diseases, physiologically or metabolically defined diseases, and aetiologically defined diseases.

Symptom diagnoses

Symptom diagnoses which are based on the presence of a single symptom represent the most primitive form of disease entity. The diagnosis 'chronic diarrhoea' may serve as an example. The definition of this disease causes no problems, as the name indicates the defining criterion. The only requirement is that we have defined what we mean by the words 'diarrhoea' and 'chronic'. General practitioners frequently use this diagnosis when they refer one of their patients to a gastroenterologist in the hope that the specialist will be able to find the cause of the patient's symptom. If the subsequent examinations show that the patient suffers from a cancer of the colon (anatomical diagnosis), ulcerative colitis (syndrome) or lactose deficiency (metabolically defined disease), then the patient receives that diagnosis instead. Symptom diagnoses are subordinate to the other types of disease entities. Sometimes, however, the specialist is not able to make a more specific diagnosis and then the patient is referred back to the general practitioner with the unchanged diagnosis 'chronic diarrhoea'. This simple example shows that symptom diagnoses are used either as preliminary diagnoses or as diagnoses made by elimination. We disregard the possibility that the specialist will not admit her ignorance and pins the unsubstantiated diagnosis 'nervous diarrhoea' on her patient.

The name of a disease may sometimes suggest that our knowledge is greater than it is. As already discussed on p. 17, the diagnosis of gastritis is used by clinicians when patients complain of upper abdominal pain for which no explanation can be found. This is a typical example of a symptom diagnosis made by elimination, but the primitive diagnosis has been disguised as an anatomically defined disease.

Some diagnoses, e.g. obesity, hypercholesterolaemia and hypertension, resemble symptom diagnoses but are based on a single clinical sign or paraclinical finding. Also in such cases the name of the disease may camouflage our ignorance, e.g. essential hypertension.

Syndromes

The general practitioner, Caleb Parry of Bath, described 'exophthalmic goitre' in 1786. Later the disease was also described by Graves (1835) in England, and by Basedow (1840) in Germany, hence the designations Graves' disease in some countries and Basedow's disease in others. Carl August Basedow was a general practitioner in Merseburg and his description is the most interesting for our purpose, as he based the diagnosis on the simultaneous presence of three clinical signs: goitre, exophthalmus and tachycardia (the so-called Merseburg triad). The relationship is shown in the diagram in Fig. 6 where

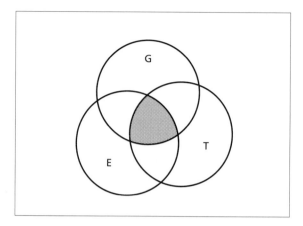

Fig. 6 The Merseburg triad. Patients with this syndrome are found in the hatched intersection of the set G (patients with goitre), the set E (patients with exophthalmus) and the set T (patients with tachycardia).

patients with 'Basedow's disease' are found in the intersection of the sets G, E and T. This triad is an example of a simple syndrome which is defined by the simultaneous presence of a fixed combination of clinical data. Later, when the function of the thyroid gland became known, this syndrome definition became obsolete, as 'Basedow's disease' was replaced by the metabolically defined disease entity, hyperthyroidism. Usually, however, disease entities defined on different levels do not delimit exactly the same patients, and that also holds true in this case. Many patients with hyperthyroidism do not fulfil Basedow's original criteria.

There are still many diseases where the pathogenesis is largely unknown, and then we still content ourselves with syndrome definitions. Ulcerative colitis is a good example. This disease name suggests that the disease entity can be defined histologically, but nevertheless pathologists will tell us that in many cases of that disease the histological picture is indistinguishable from that in other inflammatory diseases of the colon. If we make a list of all symptoms and signs found in patients who are diagnosed as having the disease, it will be found that no single symptom or sign, nor any simple combination of clinical data, fulfil the requirements of a defining criterion. However, we still have to accept the necessity of defining what is understood by this diagnosis, and therefore we must avail ourselves of a composite syndrome definition. Such a definition is illustrated by Fig. 7 [82]. The set P comprises patients who present characteristic sigmoidoscopic findings, i.e. patients with haemorrhagic proctitis; the set R comprises patients who present characteristic radiological

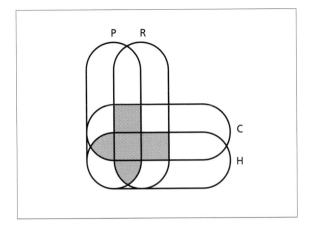

Fig. 7 Arbitrary syndrome definition of ulcerative colitis. The four sets comprise patients with characteristic sigmoidoscopic findings, i.e. proctitis (*P*), characteristic radiological findings (*R*), characteristic cytological or histological findings (*C*) and a characteristic history (*H*).

findings; the set C comprises patients with characteristic histological and cytological findings (e.g. inflammatory cells in imprints of the rectal mucosa); and the set H comprises patients presenting a characteristic history (e.g. blood in the stools). In order to make the diagnosis it is required that three of these four criteria are fulfilled, which means that the patient must belong to one of the five hatched subsets in Fig. 7.

In addition, it is required that no colonic cancer has been found which could explain the clinical picture, and that no aetiologically defined infectious disease (e.g. amoebic dysentery) has been demonstrated. Syndrome diagnoses are subordinate to anatomically defined and causally defined diseases.

This definition is not universally accepted, as clinicians elsewhere use different more or less well-defined criteria, but in some instances scientific societies have agreed on syndrome definitions in order to ensure consensus. As an example, the American Rheumatism Association [83] has proposed a syndrome definition of rheumatoid arthritis comprising the following criteria which are quoted in many textbooks:

1 morning stiffness;
2 arthritis in three or more joints;
3 arthritis in hand joints;
4 symmetric arthritis;
5 subcutaneous nodules;
6 positive reaction for rheumatoid factor; and
7 radiological changes in the joints.

Each of these criteria has been further defined, and a patient is said to suffer from rheumatoid arthritis if she fulfils at least four of these seven criteria. Other rheumatological diseases, such as systemic lupus erythematosus, have been defined in a similar manner.

Anatomically defined diseases

As a legacy of medical thinking at the beginning of the nineteenth century many disease names designate anatomical lesions. Sometimes the designation is false (e.g. gastritis) or nonspecific (e.g. ulcerative colitis), but often the anatomical lesion serves well as the defining criterion. Rectal cancer, gastric ulcer, fracture of the neck or the femur, and myocardial infarction are good examples.

From a practical point of view it is important in such cases to distinguish between two types of defining criteria. The criterion is said to be *accessible* if it is possible to ascertain, at the time of diagnosis, whether it is present or absent in a particular patient, and it is said to be *concealed* if this is not the case. A rectal cancer is accessible at proctoscopy, a gastric ulcer at gastroscopy and a hip fracture by looking at the X-ray picture. In contrast, it is not yet possible to ascertain by direct means whether or not a patient harbours a myocardial infarction, for which reason this defining criterion must be regarded as concealed. Perhaps the situation will be changed by the introduction of MR-scanning, but at present we have to rely on indirect evidence when we make or exclude this diagnosis.

If a disease is defined by a concealed criterion, it is necessary for practical purposes to supplement the theoretical definition with a *working definition*, in order to ensure maximum consensus as regards the use of the diagnostic term. Usually such working definitions take the form of a composite syndrome definition, like those mentioned above.

Some concealed criteria may be accessible in retrospect, i.e. they become accessible after the diagnostic situation. The presence of inflammation in the appendix is a concealed criterion when the diagnosis is made, but it becomes accessible when the surgeon performs a laparotomy. Similarly, the myocardial infarction becomes accessible, if the patient dies and an autopsy is made. Sometimes the anatomical defining criterion is accessible in some patients and concealed in others. It is, for instance, not always possible to prove or disprove that a patient suffers from a small pancreatic cancer.

This terminology is the key to the discussion about rational diagnosis which follows in Chapter 4.

Physiologically or metabolically defined diseases

This is a large heterogeneous group of diseases which are defined by our know-ledge of the underlying physiological or metabolic malfunction. Sometimes the defining criterion is a single clinical or paraclinical finding, such as arterial hypertension or hypercholesterolaemia. The blood pressure and the cholesterol concentration are measured on an interval scale, and the definition of the disease depends on the distinction between normal and abnormal levels.

In other cases it is much more difficult to define the disease. From a theoretical point of view it is, of course, uncontroversial to define hyperthyroidism as a disease caused by hyperfunction of the thyroid gland, diabetes mellitus as a particular disturbance of carbohydrate metabolism and bronchial asthma as bronchoconstriction mediated by an allergic reaction, but in practice these diagnoses are based on combinations of clinical data. Also in these cases we must rely on composite syndrome definitions.

Aetiologically defined diseases

This group of diseases comprises infectious diseases (e.g. typhoid fever), genetically defined, hereditary diseases (e.g. Huntington's chorea), poisonings and diseases defined by a particular environmental causal agent (e.g. asbestosis). Often the definitions combine aetiological and anatomical criteria, e.g. pneumococcal meningitis or pneumoconiosis.

Causes of disease (aetiology and pathogenesis)

According to the traditional mechanical model of disease, the clinical picture observed by the clinician is regarded as the end-result of a causal chain (Fig. 8). The disease process is elicited by a combination of genetic and environmental factors which together constitute the aetiology (from Greek *aitia* = cause). Then follows a series of changes in the organism, which may be described in physiological, biochemical, immunological or morphological terms, and collectively these changes constitute the disease mechanism or pathogenesis of the disease (*pathos* = suffering and *genesis* = generation, creation). This causal chain results in the disease, i.e. 'mechanical fault' which causes the clinical picture. Textbooks frequently contain short sections on the aetiology and pathogenesis of various diseases, but usually no sharp distinction is made between the two terms.

In order to appreciate the complexity of the causation of disease, it is

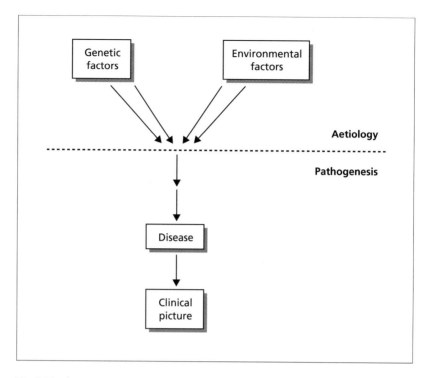

Fig. 8 The disease process.

necessary to consider briefly the concept of causality. This is a difficult topic, but for our purpose it is permissible to ignore the philosophical implications [25] and to confine ourselves to a discussion of a few simple terms. In everyday language we often say that one event X is the cause of another event Y. This wording may give the impression that an event is always caused by another single event, and to avoid that misunderstanding it is better to state that the event X is one of the factors that determine event Y. When this terminology is used it is possible to distinguish between necessary, sufficient and contributory determinants.

Factor X is a *necessary* determinant, if X always precedes Y, which of course does not imply that Y always succeeds X (Fig. 9a). We can illustrate this relationship by the determinant 'introduction into the organism of tubercle bacilli' and the effect 'pulmonary tuberculosis'. This disease is always preceded by the introduction of those bacilli, but the introduction of the bacilli does not always result in the disease. The reason for the great variation in the susceptibility of humans to infection is not fully established, but we cover up our ignorance by saying that the general resistance varies.

Pulmonary tuberculosis is a typical example of a disease about which it is

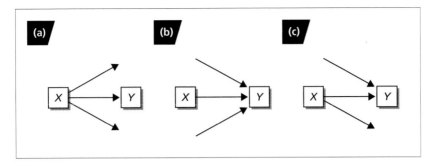

Fig. 9 Different types of causal relationships. (a) *X* is a *necessary* determinant of *Y*, as *Y* is always preceded by *X*. (b) *X* is a *sufficient* determinant of *Y*, as *X* is always succeeded by *Y*. (c) *X* is a *contributory* determinant of *Y*, as *X* is sometimes succeeded by *Y*, and *Y* is sometimes preceded by *X*.

often said that the aetiology is known or, even worse, that *the* cause is known. It would be more correct to state that a single necessary determinant has been found, but even that information is of great practical importance. The progression of the disease depends on the continued presence of the necessary determinant, and therefore elimination of the determinant will halt the disease process. Unfortunately, however, this is not the case with all diseases. We also know one necessary determinant for the development of rheumatic fever (infection with haemolytic streptococci) but the therapeutic consequence of this knowledge is smaller, as the disease may progress in spite of the elimination of the aetiological determinant.

Factor X is a *sufficient* determinant, if X is always followed by Y (Fig. 9b), which of course does not imply that Y is always preceded by X. This causal relationship can be exemplified by the determinant 'lack of iron in the food' and the effect 'anaemia'. If the body is not supplied with iron over a period of time, then anaemia is always the result, but anaemia frequently has different causes. Knowledge of a sufficient determinant may also be used therapeutically, but it is less useful from a clinical point of view. Treatment of an anaemic patient with iron will only be effective if iron deficiency is a determining factor in that particular patient. For this reason 'anaemia' is not considered a satisfactory disease entity, and it is subdivided into smaller entities, like iron-deficiency or vitamin B_{12}-deficiency anaemia, each of which is characterized by a single necessary determinant. This example also illustrates that the necessary determinant of a disease entity is not usually necessary by the grace of nature, but simply because the disease has been defined as the effect of that particular determinant.

Some determinants are neither necessary nor sufficient, but only *contributory*. This term is used if some factor X leads to an increased probability of Y, though X does not always lead to Y and Y is not always preceded by X (Fig. 9c). The logical status of contributory factors in the causal network may be difficult to define, but usually, the contributory factor is a necessary (but insufficient) component of the causal complex in a subgroup of patients with a particular disease [25,84]. Arterial hypertension, for instance, is a contributory determinant of myocardial infarction as myocardial infarction is more frequent among hypertensives than among others, and that probably means that some patients with a myocardial infarction would not have developed the disease if they had not had hypertension. There are numerous other examples of contributory factors in medicine, e.g. familial predisposition to allergic diseases, increased acid production in duodenal ulcer disease and obesity in diabetes. Knowledge of contributory determinants may sometimes be used therapeutically, as illustrated by obese patients whose diabetes respond to weight loss.

The exploration of causal relationships in clinical medicine is difficult. Often a variety of causal factors interact, or the effects are modified by feedback mechanisms which serve to maintain normal homoeostasis. Therefore, it is not surprising that the results of clinical research are often misinterpreted. Suppose, for instance, that part of the population in a developing country was immunized before it was hit by an epidemic and that the immunized persons were infected less frequently than the non-immunized ones. The most tempting conclusion is, of course, that the immunization was effective (was a contributory determinant of the prevention of infection), but there are other possible explanations. Perhaps the offer to immunize was circulated in such a way that only those people who could read were immunized and that they lived under more hygienic conditions. Then, the relationship between immunization and protection against infection might be due to a *common cause*, the higher level of education (Fig. 10a). It is also possible that those who were immunized were told at the immunization posts that they must boil all water,

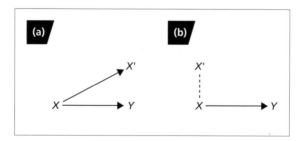

Fig. 10 Spurious relationships. (a) X' is not the cause of Y, but X' and Y have a *common* cause. (b) X' is not the cause of Y, but is a concomitant factor to X.

and that this precaution protected them against the epidemic. Then, the immunization was a *concomitant factor* to the real determining factor, the boiling of drinking water (Fig. 10b). Finally, it is possible that the observed relationship between immunization and protection against disease was a simple coincidence, i.e. that the low infection rate after immunization was due to chance.

It may also be difficult to determine what is the cause and what is the effect. When it was first found that the prevalence of *Helicobacter pylori* infection among duodenal ulcer patients is very high, it was thought by some that it was a secondary phenomenon, but now it is known that the bacillus plays a causal role, probably as a necessary (but insufficient) determinant. The interpretation of a relationship between unemployment and alcoholism is also complicated. Alcoholism may lead to unemployment, unemployment may lead to alcoholism, or the two factors may interact.

The reader of a textbook of medicine may easily get the impression that the causes of many diseases are well known, but when it is stated that the aetiology is known it usually only means that one of many aetiological factors has been isolated, and when it is stated that the pathogenesis is known, it usually only means that a few links in the chain of events leading to the observed clinical picture have been discovered. Medical scientists still find it difficult to abandon the time-honoured concept of one cause—one disease and to accept the idea of multiple determining factors. It is currently said about more and more diseases that they are 'genetic', and that may well be true in the limited sense that the genetic disposition is a contributory determinant. Usually, however, there are also environmental determinants, and it is easier to change the environment than to change the genome.

The clinical picture

The textbook describes the clinical pictures of those patients who are diagnosed as having different diseases. Thus, it will be stated in the chapter on myocardial infarction that the patients may present various symptoms (e.g. praecordial pain and anxiety), various clinical signs (tachycardia and sometimes a pericardial friction rub), and various paraclinical findings (e.g. certain electrocardiographic changes and changes in the blood concentration of different enzymes). The description of other diseases includes radiological and histological paraclinical findings such as a density on the chest X-ray in pneumonia and villous atrophy in gluten intolerance. All such clinical data are accessible, and it will often be mentioned whether they occur rarely, frequently or always in the disease in question. Other clinical data are concealed, e.g. an infarction in the mycocardium or the degeneration of the islets of Langerhans in diabetes.

The description of the disease or the nosography is not limited to a listing of the symptoms and signs. The onset, progression, possible complications and short-term prognosis of the disease are also described. Most patients, however, also wish to know to what extent a newly-diagnosed disease is likely to influence their future lives, and therefore it is unfortunate that often the textbooks provide less information about the long-term prognosis. The reason for this deficiency may well be that the textbooks are written by hospital specialists who in most cases refer their patients back to the general practitioner when the condition is stable and adequate treatment has been instituted. Some patients with chronic or recurring diseases will, of course, attend follow-up clinics at the hospital for a period of time, and others will be referred to hospital once again, if the disease takes an unexpected course, but on the whole the experience of hospital specialists, as regards the long-term prognosis of many diseases, is limited and biased. There is still a great need for clinical research where unselected groups of patients with different diseases are followed for many years. Questions about the long-term prognosis of the individual patient can, of course, only be answered in probabilistic terms, but the predictions may be more precise if they are based on prospective studies where the outcome of the disease is correlated to the patients' clinical picture at the time of diagnosis. One may, for instance, draw diagrams, like the one shown for ulcerative colitis (Fig. 7), and determine the prognosis for each subset of patients [1].

As pointed out the disease classification is a classification of patients. Each textbook chapter deals with a category of patients who are said to have a particular disease, and the reader who wishes to use that information must assume that her patients do not differ significantly from those described in the book. It cannot, however, be taken for granted that this assumption is fulfilled. The pattern of disease changes in time, due to our changing living conditions (p. 47), and the classes of patients said to suffer from particular diseases also change due to the introduction of new diagnostic methods. Therefore, the textbooks must be rewritten from time to time, but unfortunately there is considerable inertia, and, probably, most textbooks describe the disease pattern 10 or more years before the date of publication.

Geographical variation also plays an important role. It cannot be taken for granted that, for instance, European patients resemble American patients in all respects, and there are obvious problems when doctors in developing countries consult textbooks describing patients in the industrialized world.

But even within a particular society doctors must be careful when they consult their textbooks. Most textbooks are written by hospital specialists, and they do not see the same patients as general practitioners. They see different sections of the clinical spectrum.

The clinical spectrum

Arterial hypertension may serve as an example. This disease is not uncommon in hospital practice, but even more patients with this diagnosis are examined and treated in general practice. In addition, there are numerous people who fulfil the definition of the disease by having high blood pressure, who do not seek medical advice, either because they suffer no symptoms at all or because they accept their mild symptoms. Then the hypertension will only be detected if the patients see their doctor for some other reason and the doctor routinely measures the blood pressure.

Thus, a disease like hypertension presents a clinical spectrum like the one shown in Fig. 11. The spectrum comprises three types of patients with the disease:

1   non-iatrotropic cases, i.e. those cases where the patient does not seek medical advice either because she has no symptoms at all, or because the intensity of the symptoms has not reached the threshold of iatrotropy;

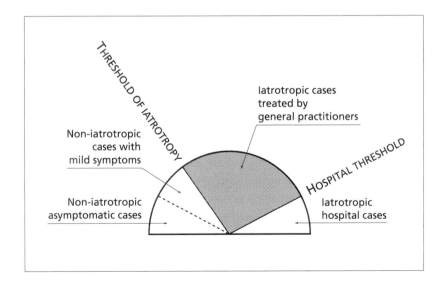

Fig. 11 The clinical spectrum.

2   iatrotropic cases which are seen by general practitioners; and

3   iatrotropic cases which have reached the hospitals.

Many diseases present such a spectrum and it is sometimes possible to distinguish between even more types of cases. In ulcerative colitis and Crohn's disease, for instance, one may also distinguish between those patients who are seen by medical gastroenterologists and those who are referred to a surgical department.

Most trials today are done at teaching hospitals, but they ought to be supplemented by clinical research in general practice, both prognostic studies and randomized clinical trials.

Diagnosis and treatment

The textbook chapters on different diseases also contain information about diagnosis and treatment. The diagnostic process and the treatment decision will be discussed in detail in the following chapters, and here we shall only make one comment. There is an increasing awareness of the need for evidence-based clinical practice which implies that the efficacy of diagnostic tests and therapeutic methods must be assessed by means of controlled clinical research. Many such studies are being done and it is surprising that the results are rarely quoted in the textbooks. The readers are rarely told anything about the rate of false positive and false negative results using different diagnostic tests, or about the therapeutic gain using different treatments. When the authors recommend different treatments they usually refer to the mechanism of action and not to the results of randomized clinical trials.

CHAPTER 4

Diagnosis

The diagnostic problem of to-day has greatly changed
–the change has come to stay;
We all have to confess, though with a sigh
On complicated tests we much rely
And use too little hand and ear and eye. [Zeta [85]]

The presentation of the diagnostic process in Chapter 1 was very brief. It was mentioned that the clinician examines his patient (collects clinical data) and then compares the patient's clinical picture with the manifestations of different diseases as they are described in the textbooks. In real life diagnostic reasoning is much more complex, and the following three patients demonstrate that it may vary from case to case.

A young man with jaundice is admitted to a teaching hospital. The consultant explains to the students that in order to make a diagnosis it is necessary to reason systematically. He tells them about the excretion of bilirubin and explains that jaundice may be caused by haemolysis, by liver-cell damage or by an occlusion of the common bile duct. He also explains which diseases may cause these disturbances and suggests what he calls a rational plan for the examination of the patient. This case illustrates the *deductive approach* to diagnosis as the clinician deduces from his pathophysiological knowledge what may be the cause of the symptom.

A middle-aged woman develops a burning pain in the left side of the chest. Inspection reveals a vesicular eruption stretching along the ribs from the spine to the sternum. The physician immediately recognizes this clinical picture and makes a diagnosis of herpes zoster. This diagnostic method may appropriately be called *pattern recognition*.

A young woman is admitted with fever and pain in the right iliac fossa associated with both direct and indirect tenderness. The surgeon knows that this clinical picture in all probability, but not with certainty, is caused by an acute appendicitis, and he decides to do a laparotomy. This is an example of *probabilistic diagnosis.*

These three types of diagnostic reasoning can, of course, rarely be isolated. The medical consultant, for instance, knew very well that haemolysis is a rare condition and that therefore this cause of jaundice is less probable than the others, and the surgeon recognized the pattern of an acute abdomen. The first part of this chapter will be devoted to probabilistic diagnosis, but later we shall consider pattern recognition and the strategy of bedside diagnosis.

The diagnostic universe

First, we shall consider the assessment of qualitative diagnostic tests, i.e. tests which provide results that are either positive or negative. The discussion of the reliability of such results requires that we distinguish between their reproducibility and their accuracy (p. 20). It was explained in Chapter 2 that the reproducibility is assessed by means of inter-observer studies and calculation of kappa values, and here we shall only consider the accuracy of the test results. The assessment of accuracy presupposes that the true diagnosis is accessible and therefore we must make the very important assumption that it is possible to establish or exclude the diagnosis with certainty by means of an independent method.

From a clinical point of view, diagnostic tests serve two different purposes. They may be used to confirm that a patient suffers from a particular disease, or they may be used to exclude that this is the case, and usually the same test does not serve both purposes equally well. Confirmation of a diagnosis requires that the positive test results are reliable, whereas exclusion of a diagnosis requires that the negative results can be relied upon.

Microscopy of the sputum for the diagnosis of pulmonary tuberculosis is a good example of a test which provides reliable positive results. The discovery of an abundance of acid-fast bacilli in the sputum leaves little doubt that the patient suffers from this disease, but, of course, the absence of bacilli does not exclude the diagnosis. A simple chest X-ray, on the other hand, provides reliable negative results. Here the probability of pulmonary tuberculosis is minimal if the films are completely normal, whereas the observation of a shadow in one of the lungs is less reliable from a diagnostic point of view, as it is often difficult to distinguish between tuberculous infiltrations and infiltrations caused by an acute pneumonia.

In most cases, however, neither the positive nor the negative test results are fully reliable. This situation may be illustrated by a simple diagram (Fig. 12) where the rectangle represents the diagnostic universe, i.e. all patients presenting a particular clinical picture. Some of the patients have a particular

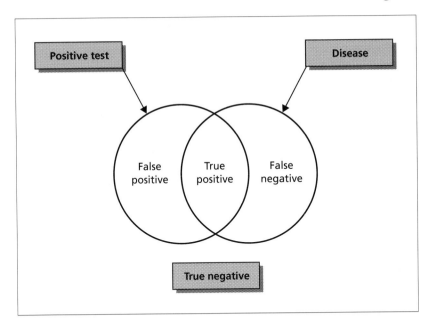

Fig. 12 The diagnostic universe.

disease (the circle to the right) and some present a positive result of the diagnostic test (the circle to the left). These two sets of patients overlap, dividing the universe into four subsets which represent patients with *true positive* results (those with a positive test who have the disease), *false positive* results (those with a positive test who do not have the disease), *true negative* results (those with a negative test who do not have the disease) and *false negative* results (those with a negative test who have the disease).

In order to assess the accuracy of the test results we must determine the number of patients in each subset, and these numbers may be recorded in a simple fourfold table (Table 5). The table shows that it is possible to calculate

Table 5 The diagnostic universe.

		Disease		
		Present	Absent	
Diagnostic test	Positive	True positives	False positives	*All positives*
	Negative	False negatives	True negatives	*All negatives*
		All with disease	*All without disease*	

the frequency of different outcomes in two ways. One may do the calculation horizontally and determine, for instance, the rate of true positive results among patients with a positive test, or one may calculate vertically and determine, for instance, the rate of true positive results among patients with the disease.

Those rates that are calculated horizontally are called *diagnostic rates*. They are the ones which the diagnostician uses when he sees the test result and wishes to determine the probability that the patient suffers from a particular disease.

Those that are calculated vertically are called *nosographic rates* as they serve to describe the disease in question. The descriptions of different diseases in medical textbooks provide nosographic information, such as information about the frequency of clinical and paraclinical findings among patients with a particular disease.

Table 5 therefore permits the calculation of the following eight different rates or probabilities. We use the generally accepted notation for conditional probabilities, according to which $P(A|B)$ means the probability of A *if* B.*

TP, FP, TN and FN in the following definitions mean true positive, false positive, true negative and false negative respectively. D + or D − mean presence or absence of disease and T + and T − mean positive or negative test.

Diagnostic probabilities

$P(D +|T +)$ = the diagnostic TP probability, i.e. the probability that a patient has the disease if the test is positive. It is calculated as: the number of true positives/total number of positives.

$P(D −|T +)$ = the diagnostic FP probability, i.e. the probability that a patient does not have the disease if the test is positive. It is calculated as: number of false positives/total number of positives.

$P(D −|T −)$ = the diagnostic TN probability, i.e. the probability that a patient does not have the disease if the test is negative. It is calculated as: number of true negatives/total number of negatives.

$P(D +|T −)$ = the diagnostic FN probability, i.e. the probability that a patient has the disease if the test is negative. It is calculated as: number of false negatives/total number of negatives.

Nosographic probabilities

$P(T +|D +)$ = the nosographic TP probability, i.e. the probability that a

---

* In order to make the presentation as simple as possible, we do not distinguish too sharply between the observed rate, referring to the sample, and the probability, referring to the population from which the sample was drawn. Later, we shall also introduce subjective probabilities.

patient with the disease has a positive test result. It is calculated as: number of true positives/total number of patients with the disease.

$P(T-|D+)$ = the nosographic FN probability, i.e. the probability that a patient with the disease has a negative test result. It is calculated as: number of false negatives/total number of patients with the disease.

$P(T-|D-)$ = the nosographic TN probability, i.e. the probability that a patient without the disease has a negative test result. It is calculated as: number of true negatives/total number of patients without disease.

$P(T+|D-)$ = the nosographic FP probability, i.e. the probability that a patient without the disease has a positive test result. It is calculated as: number of false positives/total number of patients without the disease.

The eight probabilities form four complementary pairs, e.g. the diagnostic TP rate = 1 − (the diagnostic FP probability).

Diagnosis of diseases with an accessible defining criterion

The direct method for assessing the accuracy of test results

This terminology is very useful for the assessment of the accuracy of diagnostic tests if it is possible to establish or exclude the diagnosis with certainty by means of some other method. In other words, it is required that the disease has an accessible defining criterion.

Table 6 shows the results of a study assessing the accuracy of ultrasonic scanning for the diagnosis of acute appendicitis. One hundred and eleven consecutive patients with a clinical picture suggesting this diagnosis entered the study. They

Table 6 Ultrasonography for the diagnosis of acute appendicitis. Diagnostic TP and TN rates with 95% confidence intervals are shown.

| | | Final diagnosis Appendicitis | | |
		Present	Absent	Total
Ultrasonography	Positive	42	8	50
	Negative	10	51	61
	Total	52	59	111

P(D+|T+) = 42/50 = 84.0% (70.9–92.8%)
P(D−|T−) = 51/61 = 83.6% (72.0–91.8%)

were subjected to sonography, the results of which were labelled positive or negative, and afterwards the true diagnosis was established by inspection during laparotomy. The fourfold table contains the information which is needed for estimating the diagnostic TP probability, P(D +|T +), and the diagnostic TN probability, P(D −|T −). These two probabilities are of paramount importance from a clinical point of view as P(D +|T +) tells us to which extent we may rely on the test when we wish to confirm the diagnosis whereas P(D −|T −) tells us to which extent we may rely on the test when we wish to exclude the diagnosis.

In this case the number of patients was relatively small, for which reason the calculated rates are subject to considerable uncertainty. Therefore, we have also calculated the 95% confidence intervals. This calculation will be explained in Chapter 5 (pp. 102–5), and here it is sufficient to state that we may be fairly confident that the true rate, i.e. the probability, lies within the confidence interval.

This was a very simple example, but in practice it is almost impossible to avoid methodological problems. Sometimes the diagnostic test provides ambiguous results which cannot simply be classified as positive or negative, and sometimes it proves impossible to establish the final diagnosis. Therefore, a 3 × 3 table is needed rather than a simple fourfold table.

The fourfold table in Table 6 was based on an actual study, but the recording of the results was simplified in two ways. Firstly, the uncertain results of the ultrasound scanning were recorded as positive and, secondly, those patients who did not undergo a laparotomy were classified as not having an appendicitis. Table 7

Table 7 Ultrasonography for the diagnosis of acute appendicitis. The actual results of the study are recorded in a 3 × 3 table. Some diagnostic probabilities (with 95% confidence intervals) have been calculated.

| | | Final diagnosis Appendicitis | | | |
		Present	?	Absent	*Total*
	Positive	39	4	0	*43*
Ultrasonography	?	3	1	3	*7*
	Negative	10	23	28	*61*
	Total	*52*	*28*	*31*	*111*

P(D+|T+) = 39/43 = 90.7 (77.7–97.4%)
P(D+|T?) = 3/7 = 42.9% (9.9–81.6%)
P(D−|T−) = 28/61 = 45.9% (33.1–59.2%)
P(D?|T+) = 4/43 = 9.8% (2.7–59.2%)

which summarizes the actual results [86] enables us to calculate additional conditional probabilities, such as P(D +|T?), which tells us the probability of appendicitis, if the test result is uncertain, and P(D?|T +), which shows that sometimes when the test was positive no diagnosis was made. We might also have calculated other clinically relevant diagnostic probabilities.

The method which we have described so far is called the *direct method* for the assessment of diagnostic tests, and the procedure may be summarized as follows:

1   select a sample of patients with a particular clinical picture;
2   carry out the diagnostic test and record the results;
3   establish or exclude the diagnosis by means of another method; and
4   calculate the diagnostic TP probability and the diagnostic TN probability, i.e. P(D +|T +) and P(D −|T −).

The indirect or nosographic method for assessing the accuracy of test results

Sometimes, however, a different method, which may be called the indirect or nosographic method, is recommended. Here the following procedure is used:

1   select a sample of patients with the disease and a sample of patients without the disease;
2   carry out the diagnostic test and record the results; and
3   calculate the nosographic TP probability and the nosographic TN probability, i.e. P(T +|D +) and P(T −|D −).

We may, for instance, imagine that we select 100 patients with the disease in question and 100 without it. 85 of the patients with the disease have a positive test and 95 of the patients without the disease have a negative test. Consequently, the nosographic TP probability is 85% and the nosographic TN probability is 95%. The results are shown in Table 8.

These results are only of limited value from a clinical point of view as the clinician needs to know the diagnostic probabilities. In other words, it is

Table 8 Number of positive and negative test results (T + and T−) in 100 patients with the disease (D+) and 100 patients without the disease (D−).

	D+	D−
T+	85	5
T−	15	95
Total	100	100

necessary to convert the nosographic probabilities into diagnostic probabilities. This can be done if we know the prevalence of the disease, as that information enables us to calculate the composition of the diagnostic universe. If, for instance, the prevalence of the disease is 10% we may imagine a diagnostic universe comprising 100 patients with the disease (of whom 85% have a positive test) and 900 patients without the disease (of whom 95% have a negative test). This hypothetical example leads to the fourfold table shown as Table 9a which permits a calculation of the relevant diagnostic probabilities. It is seen that the test is only moderately reliable for making the diagnosis as no more

Table 9 The diagnostic universe corresponding to the figures in Table 8, if the prevalence of the disease is (a) 10%, (b) 1%, and (c) 80%. Same notation as in Table 8.

(a)

	D+	D−	Total
T+	85	45	130
T−	15	855	870
Total	100	900	

P(D+|T+) = 85/130 = 65.4%
P(D−|T−) = 855/870 = 98.3%

(b)

	D+	D−	Total
T+	85	495	580
T−	15	9405	9420
Total	100	9900	

P(D+|T+) = 85/580 = 14.7%
P(D−|T−) = 9405/9420 = 99.8%

(c)

	D+	D−	Total
T+	85	1	86
T−	15	24	39
Total	100	25	

P(D+|T+) = 85/86 = 98.8%
P(D−|T−) = 24/39 = 61.5%

than 65.4% of those patients who have a positive test also have the disease, whereas it is much more useful for excluding the diagnosis as 98.3% of the patients with a negative test do not have the disease.

We could also imagine that the prevalence was no more than 1%. This is also a realistic possibility as sometimes we wish to rule out improbable diagnoses. In that case we should need 9900 patients to balance the 100 patients with the disease and the result of the calculations are shown in Table 9b. Then the test would be useless for establishing the diagnosis as a little less than 15% of patients with a positive test would have the disease, but the reliability of negative test results would be even higher than in the previous example.

Table 9c represents the other extreme. Here the prevalence is 80% which is realistic when we were dealing with a clinical picture that is highly suggestive of one particular disease. Now the test is reliable for confirming the diagnosis as $P(D+|T+)$ is almost 99%, but quite unreliable for excluding the diagnosis, $P(D-|T-)$ being 61.5%.

It is, however, not necessary to construct a fictitious diagnostic universe in order to convert nosographic into diagnostic probabilities. It may also be done by means of Bayes' theorem which in its simplest form looks like this:

$$P(D+|T+) = P(T+|D+)\frac{P(D+)}{P(T+)}$$

In this formula $P(D+)$ is the unconditional probability that a patient from this diagnostic universe has the disease, i.e. the disease prevalence, and $P(T+)$ is the unconditional probability that a patient from the universe has a positive test. Usually, $P(T+)$ is not known, but then one may use the following more complex formula (where $P(T+)$ is calculated from the available information):

$$P(D+|T+) = \frac{P(T+|D+)P(D+)}{P(T+|D+)P(D+)+(1-P(T+|D+))(1-P(D+))}$$

The following calculation of $P(D+|T+)$, which refers to the first of the examples, gives exactly the same result as before (Table 9a):

$$P(D+|T+) = \frac{0.85\times0.10}{0.85\times0.10+0.05\times0.90} = 0.654$$

$P(D-|T-)$ can be calculated by a similar formula (replacing + by – and vice versa).

The indirect or nosographic method has been discussed in some detail as it illustrates well that the value of the diagnostic probabilities depends on two factors: the nosographic probabilities and the prevalence of the disease. As we shall explain below, Bayesian reasoning is required whenever we wish to use nosographic knowledge (textbook knowledge) for diagnostic purposes.

However, the formal use of the indirect method for the assessment of diagnostic tests is rarely warranted. The procedure suggests that one may determine the nosographic probabilities in one diagnostic universe and then use that information to calculate the diagnostic probabilities in another universe, if only one takes into account the prevalence of the disease. That, however, is not permissible as both the nosographic probabilities and the prevalence differ in different clinical settings. The assessment of a diagnostic test must be confined to one well-defined diagnostic universe. It cannot be taken for granted, for instance, that ultrasound scanning is equally effective for confirming or excluding a diagnosis of pancreatic cancer in patients presenting with abdominal pain, patients presenting with jaundice, and patients presenting with a palpable mass in the abdomen. We must assume that the frequency of positive results among patients with the disease (the nosographic TP rate) differs in these three groups of patients. Similarly, it cannot be assumed that ultrasound scanning is equally effective in general practice as in hospital practice. General practitioners wish to diagnose the early stages of the disease and the small tumours in such patients are more likely to be missed by the ultrasound scan than the larger tumours seen by hospital specialists.

Therefore, it only makes limited sense to discuss in general terms whether or not a particular test is good or bad for diagnosing a particular disease. Usually, one can only tell whether or not the test results are sufficiently accurate either for confirming the diagnosis or for excluding the diagnosis in patients who present a particular clinical picture and who belong to a particular part of the clinical spectrum of the disease.

In other words, we cannot assess a diagnostic test unless we define in advance the diagnostic universe and, when that has been done, it is usually just as easy to select one random sample of patients belonging to that universe and determine directly the diagnostic TP and TN rates. It is simply a waste of time to determine the nosographic probabilities and the prevalence, and then calculate the diagnostic probabilities. The indirect method is only a realistic alternative if the disease is very rare, as in that case the determination of the diagnostic TP rate, using the direct method, may require a very large sample of patients.

There is an increasing interest in the assessment of diagnostic tests, but there is a need for many more studies. The resources of most health services are limited and, whenever possible, we ought to assess the accuracy of the new, sometimes very costly, diagnostic techniques before they find their way to the daily routine. It is also to be hoped that the results of the assessments will find their way to the standard textbooks of medicine, which today contain little precise information about the value of different tests.

Undoubtedly, many diagnostic tests are much overrated. Gastroenterologists pay much attention to the appearance of the mucosa during gastroduodenoscopy, but a Norwegian population survey of endoscopic and histological findings in subjects with and without dyspepsia revealed that only 10% in both groups had what was considered a normal mucosa. The endoscopic findings, with the possible exceptions of peptic ulcer disease and endoscopic duodenitis, showed no association of clinical value with dyspepsia [87].

Terminological confusion

The terminology that has been introduced in this chapter is not generally accepted. The authors of most textbooks on clinical epidemiology and most papers dealing with diagnostic problems write about the specificity and sensitivity of diagnostic tests and the predictive value of positive and negative test results. These terms (which we shall refer to as the 'international terminology') are defined as follows using our terminology:

Specificity = nosographic TN rate = $P(T-|D-)$

Sensitivity = nosographic TP rate = $P(T+|D+)$

Predictive value of positive test (PV_{pos}) = diagnostic TP rate = $P(D+|T+)$

Predictive value of negative test (PV_{neg}) = diagnostic TN rate = $P(D-|T-)$

Terminological problems are, of course, not very interesting *per se* and one may argue that it does not really matter which words we use. In this case, however, the commonly used terms invite misunderstandings.

Only those who have a very good grasp of diagnostic logic will appreciate that in the international terminology the terms specificity and sensitivity have been redefined so that they no longer have the same meaning as in ordinary language. If you say, for instance, that a blood test is very specific, you usually mean that you can rely on the positive test results as there will only be few false positive results. In other words, according to the ordinary use of the word, a specific test is a test where the diagnostic TP rate is high, but in the international terminology the specificity is defined as the nosographic TN rate. This is obviously a source of confusion as a high nosographic TN rate need not be associated with a high diagnostic TP rate. In one of the examples above (Table 9b) the specificity (using the international definition) was 95%, but the diagnostic TP rate was only about 15%.

Similarly, when we say that a blood test is very sensitive, we usually mean that we can rely on the negative results, i.e. that it rarely fails when the blood contains the substance in question. In other words, according to ordinary usage, a sensitive test is a test where the diagnostic TN rate is high, but in the international terminology it is defined as the nosographic TP rate. That may also lead to misunderstandings. In Table 9c the nosographic TP rate was 85%, but the diagnostic TN rate only about 62%.

Frequently it is also suggested that the specificity and sensitivity (i.e. the nosographic probabilities) are stable measures of the reliability of a diagnostic test whereas the diagnostic probabilities are unstable as they depend on the prevalence of the disease. It is this idea which invites the misconception that one may determine the sensitivity and specificity in one clinical setting and then use these results to calculate the diagnostic probabilities for other clinical settings, taking into account the varying prevalence of the disease. As we have explained already this procedure is not acceptable as nosographic rates, as well as diagnostic rates, depend on the diagnostic universe.

It is also unfortunate that the terms diagnostic and nosographic rates or probabilities have no equivalents in the standard terminology. The false positive rate is a commonly used term, but it is rarely stated how it is calculated, i.e. whether it is the diagnostic or the nosographic FP rate. Many clinicians who hear that the false positive rate is only 5% will believe that then there is only a 5% chance that a patient with a positive test does not have the disease in question and, if the rate is nosographic, that may be a grave misunderstanding. We may again refer to Table 9b where the nosographic FP rate was 5% while the diagnostic FP rate was about 85%.

The nosographic rates are of little interest when the clinician seeks the right diagnosis in one of his patients, but they may serve other purposes. Those who plan mass screening for some disease must take into account both the nosographic TP rate and the nosographic FP rate. The former supplies the information how many people with the disease are caught in the net, and the latter how many persons without the disease are also caught. But the interpretation of a test result in the individual case still requires diagnostic thinking. Most people will be impressed when they hear that the sensitivity and specificity of a test used for mass screening are both 98%, but if the prevalence is only 1 per 1000 (which is not unrealistic in a screening project) there is a 95% probability that a patient with a positive test does not have the disease.

The international terminology refers to the diagnostic rates as the predictive values of the test, the predictive value of a positive test being the diagnostic TP rate and the predictive value of a negative test being the diagnostic TN rate. That also serves to muddle the discussion. These expressions originated in epidemiology where it is reasonable to talk about the predictive value of different risk factors, but they make no sense in a diagnostic context. Prediction (foretelling) implies reasoning from a causal factor to some possible future effect, but that is not the case when a clinician makes a diagnosis. He analyses the patient's clinical picture and seeks the cause of the observed symptoms and signs; he reasons from effect to cause, not from cause to effect.

The present terminological and conceptual confusion may well explain that few clinicians have a good grasp of diagnostic logic.

Quantitative data

So far we have only considered the assessment of qualitative tests, but many of those diagnostic tests which are used in everyday clinical practice are quantitative. Clinicians, however, do not always quote the exact results when they discuss their patients, but confine themselves to stating that the patient has a low serum potassium, a normal alkaline phosphatase or eosinophilia. They reduce the level of measurement from an interval scale to an ordinal or binary scale, and that, of course, raises the question how one distinguishes between normal and abnormal (high or low) test results.

Suppose that we wish to assess the value of a quantitative test for the diagnosis of an anatomically defined disease. The reader can probably find an example within his own sphere of interest, e.g. serum alkaline phosphatase for the diagnosis of obstructive jaundice, α-fetoprotein for the diagnosis of hepatocellular carcinoma, or urine catecholamines for the diagnosis of phaeochromocytoma. First, a number of patients suspected of having the disease are collected, then the patients are subjected to the new test and, finally, the true diagnosis is established. Figure 13 shows what the results may look like when the assessment is made of a quantitative blood analysis, the unit of measurement being mmol/L. The histogram pointing upwards shows the distribution of patients who were found not to suffer from the disease in question, and the histogram pointing downwards shows the distribution of

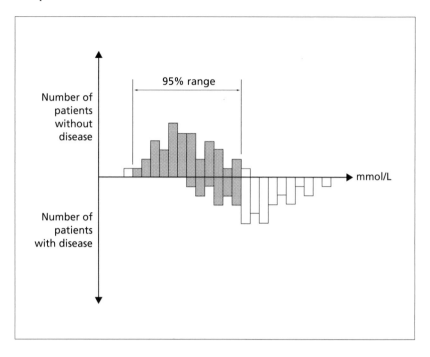

Fig. 13 The histogram pointing downwards shows the distribution of the results of a diagnostic test in patients suffering from a particular disease. The histogram pointing upwards shows the distribution in patients not suffering from the disease.

patients with the disease. For the sake of simplicity we assume that patients without the disease give the same results as normal subjects, and in that case the observed 95% range which is shown in the figure is the same as the normal range. It is seen that the new test tends to give higher results in patients with the disease than in patients without the disease, but there is a considerable overlap.

We now wish to draw a line separating normal from high values, assuming that abnormally low values have no clinical significance, and this distinction can be made at different levels. Traditionally, one would prefer to draw the line at the upper limit of the 95% range, and that has been done in Fig. 14a where the histogram for the sake of clarity has been drawn as a continuous curve. By means of the abscissa axis and the vertical line through the upper limit of the normal range, the patients have been divided into four groups.

The upper left quadrant contains those patients who gave a true negative result as the result was negative and the patients did not have the disease. The

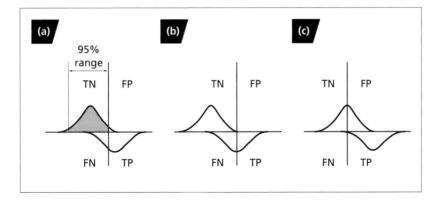

Fig. 14 (a) Conventional distinction between normal and elevated values. (b) Distinction between normal and elevated values which eliminates false positive results. (c) Distinction between normal and elevated values which eliminates false negative results. For the sake of simplicity the histograms have been drawn as continuous curves. TN = true negative results, FP = false positive results, FN = false negative results, TP = true positive results.

upper right quadrant contains those patients who gave a false positive result, and they constitute 2.5% of all patients without the disease, as the 95% normal range cuts off the 2.5% highest and the 2.5% lowest values. The lower left quadrant contains the patients with false negative results, and the true positive results are found in the lower right quadrant.

It is also possible to draw the line between normal and elevated values at other levels. In Fig. 14b the distinction is made in such a way that all patients without the disease are said to give a normal test result. In that case there will be no false positive results, but in return a large number of patients with the disease present a false negative result.

In Fig. 14c we have gone to the other extreme as the line has been drawn in such a way that the test result is said to be elevated in all patients with the disease. Now there are no false negative, but many false positive results.

It is also relevant in this case to distinguish between diagnostic and nosographic probabilities. In Fig. 14a the number of patients who gave false positive results (the patients in the upper right quadrant) constituted 2.5% of all patients without the disease (all results above the line) and therefore 2.5% is the nosographic FP rate. If instead the number of false positive results is related to the total number of positive results (all results to the right of the vertical line), we shall obtain the diagnostic FP rate.

The example shows that it is possible in theory to adjust the diagnostic rates to fit the problem at hand, and that also applies to some descriptive qualitative tests. It is, for instance, not possible to distinguish sharply between benign cells and malignant cells in cytological preparations, and by altering the criteria it may be possible to alter the proportion of false positives and false negatives. Stringent criteria give few false positive results and many false negatives, whereas less stringent criteria have the opposite effect [88].

These examples illustrate that no clear-cut distinction can be made between quantitative and qualitative data. Classification of cells as malignant or benign is from a formal point of view a binary scale measurement, but nevertheless there is a gradual transition between the two classes, and it is up to the cytologist to draw the line between them. The potassium concentration of serum is measured on an interval scale, but the physician has to reduce the measurement to a lower level in order to decide if a patient suffers from hyperkaliaemia, has a normal concentration, or suffers from hypokaliaemia. The clinician is a decision-maker and before he can take further action he must, as it was once said, choose his operating points on the criterion axis [2].

Up to now we have only considered the diagnostic importance of single tests, but that is an over-simplification of clinical decision-making. The physician who sees a jaundiced patient will be interested in both the alkaline phosphatase and the aminotransferase. If the aminotransferase level is highly elevated and the alkaline phosphatase is only slightly increased, infectious hepatitis is suspected, and if the opposite is true obstructive jaundice is more likely. Here the physician uses the combination of two quantitative paraclinical findings which have been reduced to an ordinal scale with three classes (normal, slightly elevated, highly elevated), but usually diagnostic reasoning is much more complicated.

Diagnosis of diseases with a concealed defining criterion

So far the value of diagnostic tests has been discussed in probabilistic terms. Usually, we cannot guard ourselves against false positive and false negative results in the individual case, but, according to the probabilistic approach, we should attempt to determine the probability that the test results are correct. This approach was illustrated by a number of numerical examples, but they were all based on the assumption that the truth of the diagnosis could be established by independent means. This assumption, however, is rarely fulfilled in practice, and in actual fact we have only been dealing with ideal cases. If the disease has a concealed defining criterion, the true diagnosis may never be revealed, and in clinical syndromes, as we shall explain later, the truth of the diagnosis is almost a matter of opinion.

Myocardial and pulmonary infarction are typical examples of diseases with a concealed defining criterion. A textbook author once wrote that the discovery of increased concentrations of some enzymes in patients with myocardial infarction 'ushered in a new era of diagnostic accuracy' and the same could have been said about the introduction of pulmonary scintigraphy for the diagnosis of infarctions in the lungs. We do not, of course, wish to contest the justification of such statements, but on reflection it will be found that they are not quite as simple as they sound. Imagine, for instance, that we wanted to assess the diagnostic accuracy of an elevated MB (myocardial band) isoenzyme of creatine phosphokinase for diagnosing myocardial infarction. According to the direct method, the procedure would be as follows: first, some patients are selected who are suspected of having a myocardial infarction, for instance patients who developed sudden praecordial pain. Next, the serum content of the enzyme is determined, and a distinction is made between a normal and an elevated concentration. Then, however, we run into difficulties, as fortunately most of the patients survive, and in all those cases we shall not know with absolute certainty whether or not the patient had an infarction, and therefore we shall never learn whether the test result was true or false. It is impossible to calculate the diagnostic TP and TN rates, if the defining criterion remains concealed, and instead it is necessary to substantiate the accuracy of the test results by indirect means. This can be done in a number of different ways.

Firstly, we may rely on our knowledge of anatomy and physiology and of the pathogenesis of the disease. We know that the heart muscle is damaged by the blocked blood flow and we understand that this may have the effect that enzymes normally found in the heart leak into the blood. We also know that the MB-isoenzyme is found only in the heart whereas other isoenzymes of creatine phosphokinase are also present in skeletal muscle. Therefore, it is reasonable to expect that the diagnostic TP rate will be higher if we only determine the MB-isoenzyme. However, we must ascertain that the laboratory techniques which are used for isolating the isoenzyme are sufficiently specific.

Similarly, we may deduce from our theoretical knowledge that combined pulmonary perfusion and ventilation scintigraphy is a useful test. We shall not go into details, but just sketch the flow of the reasoning. The technetium[99m]-labelled albumin macroaggregates which are infused are caught in the pulmonary capillary bed, and normally the scintigram exhibits a homogeneous distribution of radioactivity in the lungs. In pulmonary infarction, however, the blood flow to a section of the lung will be blocked, and a 'defect' with absent radioactivity will be seen. Therefore, it is assumed that the diagnostic TN probability is high, but it is not assumed that the diagnostic TP probability is also high, as other lung diseases may also cause local disturbances of the blood flow. To solve this problem a ventilation test is done where the patient inhales a radioactive gas. Pulmonary embolism does not reduce the ventilation of the affected zone and therefore the ventilation scintigram will be normal. Consequently, the two tests are interpreted together and it is assumed that the diagnostic TP probability is high, if the perfusion scan is positive and the ventilation scan negative.

It is this kind of reasoning which has led to the introduction of these and many other tests, and although the flow of the arguments may seem very logical, they only provide sophisticated circumstantial evidence. In the case of pulmonary scintigraphy, we cannot be sure that small infarctions are always detected or that the ventilation scan is always normal in other diseases, and we know that the inter-observer variation may be considerable (p. 26). Therefore, there can be little doubt that in clinical practice we encounter both false positive and false negative results, but since the defining criterion in most cases remains concealed, we do not know how often this happens.

If the patient dies and an autopsy is performed, the defining criterion becomes accessible, and usually the diagnosis which was made when the patient was alive is confirmed. Then it is tempting to conclude that the results of the test are also accurate in those patients who survive, but that is of course not certain. Patients may die from a myocardial or a pulmonary infarction, but perhaps the fatality rate of those conditions that mimic these diseases clinically is low, and in that case the false positive results will not be detected at the autopsy table.

Extrapolation from patients who die to patients who survive was first introduced by the French pathologists at the beginning of the nineteenth century (p. 42), and it was also used by With in his treatize on gastric ulcer in 1881 (p. 47). He observed that those young women who were admitted because of an acute abdominal crisis, and died, had a gastric ulcer, and since many of them presented a history of epigastric pain he assumed that other young women with epigastric pain also had a gastric ulcer. He was probably right, but it cannot be proved.

We do not, however, wish to imply that observations made at the autopsy table are of little interest. On the contrary, they are very important as they serve to confront the clinician with his diagnostic mistakes. Until a few decades ago autopsies were done almost routinely in many European countries. Every time a patient died the clinicians who had treated the patient visited the pathology department and inspected the organs. Now, for a number of reasons, the autopsy rate has dropped drastically, which must mean that some diagnostic errors never come to light. This may enhance clinicians' tendency to overestimate the accuracy of the tests which they use.

Sometimes when it is not possible to establish the diagnosis with certainty, it is decided to circumvent the problems by choosing a gold standard. In other words, the results of the new test are compared with the results of some other test which is considered reliable, but may have the disadvantage that it is more expensive or unpleasant for the patients. There are, for instance, a number of studies where the results of pulmonary scintigraphy are compared with the results of pulmonary angiography. This is not an unreasonable idea, but it is far from certain that the reliability of angiography is perfect, as regards reproducibility and accuracy. If the result of one method is positive and that of the other negative, it is not certain which is correct and which is wrong.

The course of the disease and the combined results of other tests may also provide a gold standard. This procedure was used in the case of the MB-isoenzyme. This test is considered useful for establishing or excluding the diagnosis of a myocardial infarction at a very early stage, and its reliability for that purpose could be assessed by relating the results to the final diagnosis after prolonged observation of the symptoms, the ECG-changes and the changes of the levels of other enzymes [89].

In practice, the diagnosis of diseases with a concealed defining criterion also involves simple pattern recognition. Clinicians may regard the diseases as clinical syndromes, which means that they take into account all the clinical data, including symptoms, signs and paraclinical findings, and make the diagnosis if the total clinical picture is sufficiently typical. If, however, diagnosis is viewed from this angle, we face other equally difficult problems.

Syndrome diagnosis

Many years ago, at a clinical conference, a chemical pathologist proposed a new serological test for the diagnosis of infectious mononucleosis. He said (we cannot remember the exact figures) that Paul Bunnel's test, which was the only one used at that time, was positive only in 70% of cases, whereas the new test was positive in 90% of cases. A critical clinician pondered over this information and replied rather unkindly: 'If it is possible to calculate these percentages, then there must be a third method by which the diagnosis can be made with 100% certainty. We should like to hear more about this third method and discuss its introduction.' There was, of course, no such method, as infectious mononucleosis at that time (before the importance of Epstein–Barr virus was recognized) must be regarded as an undefined, or at most arbitrarily defined, clinical syndrome, and the percentages mentioned did not prove the superiority of the new test.

One might also have raised another equally justified objection. The quoted percentages represent nosographic TP rates, and as explained above it is necessary to determine also the nosographic TN rate, and especially the relevant diagnostic rates.

A paper was published recommending a new method of diagnosing hyperthyroidism [90] in much the same manner. The author had collected a group of patients in whom the diagnosis had been made using all available diagnostic tests, including the new one. He then calculated which test was positive in the greatest number of cases, and *mirabile dictu* the new test won the competition. The only conclusion which can be drawn from such a study is that the author attached more importance to the results of the new test than to the results of the others, when he made the diagnosis. It is important that the consumer of medical literature is not deceived when medical writers use circular arguments.

Doctors still make similar mistakes as they have little training in analysing such logical problems of syndrome diagnosis (including metabolically defined diseases which are treated like clinical syndromes), but it is much easier to criticize than to be constructive. Where clinical syndromes are concerned it is difficult to lay down clear-cut principles for the assessment of new diagnostic methods.

One may say that syndrome diagnosis is simply a problem of pattern recognition. If we assume that all common syndromes are well defined, the diagnosis of a syndrome simply consists of the demonstration of those clinical data which must be present according to the syndrome definition. According to this point of view, the diagnostic tests only serve to fill in the patient's clinical picture, and it has little meaning to discuss the probability of the diagnosis. If, for instance, a patient fulfils the criteria of rheumatoid arthritis mentioned on p. 53, then he has got the disease, and if he does not fulfil the criteria he has not got the disease. It is a case of all or nothing and not a question of probabilities.

This presentation, however, oversimplifies matters, because in everyday clinical medicine syndrome diagnosis undoubtedly includes a probabilistic element.

When the clinician has recorded his patient's iatrotropic symptoms and the usual routine data, he will consider which diagnosis is the most probable, and if this diagnosis is a clinical syndrome, he will institute those investigations which are necessary to fill in the clinical picture. If the patient does not fulfil the criteria for that syndrome, he will then institute those investigations which are needed to make or exclude the second most probable disease, and so on.

Most syndromes, however, are not well defined, and even if they were, there would still be patients who would only fulfil some of the criteria for that particular syndrome. When that is the case the clinician must decide if he still wants to make the diagnosis, i.e. if he still wants to treat the patient as if all the criteria were fulfilled. It is, for instance, not unusual at a rheumatological department that a patient is thought to have a so-called connective tissue disease, although the serological reactions and the skin and muscle biopsies have not provided results which fulfil all the accepted diagnostic criteria for any syndrome belonging to that group of diseases. In such a case it may still be reasonable to start treatment with corticosteroids, because it is considered probable that the patient has a connective tissue disease after all, which really means that probably the patient will respond to treatment in the same way as those patients who fulfil all the criteria.

It is important to understand how syndromes are first described, and how they change. Rheumatoid arthritis may again serve as an example as we still do not know enough about the disease mechanisms to be able to suggest a pathogenetic or an aetiological definition.

This syndrome was originally introduced because clinicians had observed patients with clinical pictures which resembled each other to such an extent that it was considered justified to say that they had the same disease. Such clinical pictures characterized by symptoms and clinical signs formed the original nucleus of the syndrome, and the patients in question may be regarded as 'typical' cases of rheumatoid arthritis. They are represented by the circular area *A* in Fig. 15a. In addition, 'atypical' cases were observed, i.e. patients whose clinical pictures to a varying extent differed from the 'typical' pictures. If the difference was small, the patients were still said to have rheumatoid arthritis (the annular area *B* in Fig. 15a), and if the difference was larger this diagnosis was not made (area *C* in Fig. 15a). Thus, the final result is that the hatched area of the figure comprises patients who were given the diagnosis of rheumatoid arthritis. The boundary between these categories of patients was of course not sharp, but the example serves to illustrate the principles of syndrome diagnosis on purely clinical criteria.

In the 1930s it was discovered that serum from patients with rheumatoid arthritis frequently contained agglutinins against haemolytic streptococci,

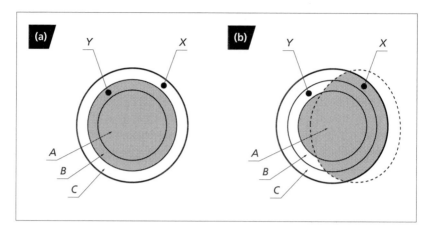

Fig. 15 Diagnosis of rheumatoid arthritis before (a) and after (b) the introduction of a serological diagnostic test. See text for further explanation. X and Y represent two patients whose diagnosis was affected by the introduction of the test.

and the agglutination reaction became accepted as a diagnostic test. The resulting influence on the diagnosis of the syndrome is shown in Fig. 15b, in which the oval figure represents all patients with a positive test.

Patients with typical clinical pictures (area *A*) still received the diagnosis of rheumatoid arthritis, since it may be presumed that a negative result of the new test would not make the clinician reject the diagnosis when the clinical evidence was strong. In patients with atypical pictures (areas *B* and *C*), however, the test must have influenced the diagnosis, because it was in these cases that the clinician needed the additional paraclinical evidence. If he relied on the test, which he probably did as he used it, we may presume that he made a diagnosis of rheumatoid arthritis if the test was positive and that he did not make the diagnosis if it was negative. The situation is illustrated by Fig. 15b, where the hatched area shows which patients were labelled as having rheumatoid arthritis after the introduction of the test. The net result simply was that the use of the diagnostic term had changed.

Since then this test has become obsolete, but others have replaced it as diagnostic aids, and one may assume that each time the syndrome diagnosis was affected. This situation was foreseen by the American Rheumatism Association. When they first established a set of criteria they commented that it must be revised from time to time so that the definition does not become outdated [91].

This example admittedly represents armchair reasoning but it illustrates the fundamental difference between the use of diagnostic tests in clinical syndromes and in, for instance, anatomically defined diseases with an accessible defining criterion. We cannot assess the tests that we use for the diagnosis of clinical syndromes by quoting the diagnostic TP and TN rates as we ourselves determine the accuracy of the results. If we usually make the diagnosis when the test is positive and usually exclude the diagnosis when the test is negative, we shall of course find that the diagnostic rates are high. Many tests used in the daily routine have probably been introduced in this dubious manner, and once they have been accepted we soon feel that we cannot do without them.

The introduction of new tests may be prompted by our more or less well-founded hypotheses about the aetiology and pathogenesis of the disease, but we must always ask ourselves if they are really necessary. Unnecessary changes of the diagnostic criteria have the unfortunate consequence that past clinical experience may become outdated. If the current diagnostic criteria no longer correspond to those entry criteria which were used in a large randomized trial, the results of that trial may become less useful for clinical purposes.

Three patients

The analysis of the diagnostic decision on the preceding pages may be summarized by means of three clinical cases where two skilled clinicians disagree about the diagnosis.

The first patient is admitted with an acute abdomen. One clinician believes that the patient has an acute appendicitis whereas his colleague does not think that this is the case. Here, one clinician is right and the other is wrong, and if they agree on doing a laparotomy and open the patient's abdomen we shall soon find out who is right and who is wrong. The defining criterion becomes accessible at the operation.

The second patient suddenly developed praecordial pain. All the necessary investigations are done, including ECGs and enzyme tests, but the two clinicians read the evidence differently. One believes that the patient has a myocardial infarction and the other does not think so. In this case, too, one clinician must be right and the other wrong, but if the patient gets well and is discharged from hospital some days later we shall never learn the truth. The defining criterion remains concealed.

The third patient has a complex clinical picture with muscular weakness and a skin eruption. The necessary investigations are done, including skin and muscle biopsies. One clinician believes that it is a case of dermatomyositis, while the other denies this. In this case it makes little sense to say that one is right and the other wrong, as dermatomyositis is a clinical syndrome for which no generally accepted set of diagnostic criteria exists. We must simply conclude that these two rheumatologists define the syndrome differently. They may, however, decide to see the patient at regular intervals, and if the patient later develops a clinical picture which is so typical that it is recognized by everybody, we may conclude in retrospect which rheumatologist made the right diagnosis.

These three patients summarize the fundamental logical problems which we face whenever we try to assess the accuracy of the diagnostic methods which we use. Stringent criteria have been worked out for testing new treatments (Chapter 6), but such criteria are missing for assessing new diagnostic methods. A recent survey revealed that only a small minority of papers dealing with the assessment of diagnostic methods were methodologically acceptable [92], and every week critical readers of medical journals may find examples of studies which are heavily biased in one way or another, which exhibit circular logic, misinterpret the calculated probabilities or ignore patients with uncertain test results. Typically, the indirect method is used and only the nosographic probabilities (sensitivity and specificity) are quoted, even in diseases such as temporal arteritis [93] where information about the diagnostic FN probability is essential due to the dire consequences of missing the diagnosis.

Some of the problems reflect the nature of the disease classification, but in those cases where it is impossible to establish the truth of the test results, we should remember that the diagnosis is not an end in itself. The diagnostic decision is only, as it was once said, a mental resting place on the way to treatment. If we accept this way of thinking, the truth of the diagnosis becomes less important, and we may instead try to assess whether the introduction of the new test improves the treatment results. Years ago, before the routine use of pulmonary scintigraphy for the diagnosis of pulmonary infarction, one might have done a large randomized clinical trial (Chapter 6) of patients with clinical pictures suggesting this diagnosis. Then treatment in one group might be instituted on the basis of the clinical findings and in the other on the basis of the scintigrams and the clinical findings. If the patients in the latter group fared better, one would have proved that the introduction of this diagnostic procedure was beneficial. Otherwise, it would have been shown to be superfluous.

Diagnosis in practice

Frequential and subjective probabilities

In this chapter we have repeatedly used the words probabilistic and probability. In the numerical example in Table 9a (p. 70) the diagnostic TP probability was 65.4% and the diagnostic TN probability was 98.3%. Later, it was stated that there might be a 95% probability that an individual taking part in a screening project does not have the disease, in spite of the fact that the test result is positive (p. 75), and it was mentioned in connection with syndrome diagnosis that the clinician facing an individual patient must always consider the probability of different diagnostic options (p. 82).

These statements may seem quite straightforward, but in fact they represent two very different probability concepts as the diagnostic probabilities in the first two statements refer to groups of patients, whereas the probabilities in the last two statements refer to individual patients [4]. We shall briefly consider this theoretical question as it serves to clarify a fundamental problem in evidence-based clinical medicine. It helps to explain what it means to make decisions about the individual patient on the basis of experience which has been gained by studying groups of patients.

When we talk about diagnostic or nosographic probabilities we use the traditional frequential or statistical probability concept as the probability represents the 'true' frequency in the population. If we say, for instance, that the diagnostic TP probability is 80%, we mean that the frequency of patients with the disease is 80% in a population of persons with a positive test. In practice, we can, of course, only determine the diagnostic TP rate (or frequency) in a limited sample of patients, but for the sake of simplicity we take it for granted in this discussion that the sample is so large that we can ignore the difference between the observed and the true rate.

If, however, we say that there is an 80% probability that a particular patient has the disease, we must mean something else. It cannot be a frequency as it makes no sense to say that the frequency of the disease in one patient is 80%. The patient either has or does not have the disease. Here we use the subjective probability concept where the probability expresses our degree of confidence in the presence or absence of a particular phenomenon. When we say that there is an 80% probability that a patient suffers from a particular disease, we mean that we are 80% confident that this is the case.

Our justification for that degree of confidence may well be that we have read a paper in a medical journal which reported that the diagnostic TP rate among patients presenting similar clinical pictures was 80%, and in that case the argument goes as follows: the subjective probability of (our confidence in) the diagnosis in this patient is 80% as the frequential probability of the diagnosis among similar patients with a positive test is 80%.

This analysis may seem pedantic, but it is important, as it leaves room for the individualization of clinical reasoning. Perhaps the clinician possesses additional information about the patient. There may have been other cases of the disease in the family, and if it is known to be hereditary he might conclude that in this particular case his confidence in the diagnosis is not 80%, but 95%.

The subjective probability concept is of particular interest when we are dealing with diseases with a concealed defining criterion. Imagine a physician who sees a patient with symptoms suggesting pulmonary embolism whose pulmonary scintigraphy shows the typical 'mismatch' between the perfusion and ventilation scans. He will say that there is almost a 100% probability that this patient has a pulmonary infarction, but this time the subjective probability is not based on an observed frequency as in most cases the diagnosis remains concealed. His confidence in the diagnosis is based on knowledge of the pathogenesis of the disease and the theoretical rationale of the two forms of scintigraphy.

Diagnostic strategy

We should have liked to explain in detail how clinicians think when they examine their patients and seek the right diagnosis, but unfortunately nobody has ever been able to do so. Diagnostic reasoning is extremely complex, and we shall only be able to discuss this topic in general terms.

The clinician starts thinking about the diagnosis as soon as he has seen the patient and the patient has revealed his complaints (the iatrotropic symptoms). In some cases he will immediately make a diagnosis by simple pattern recognition (e.g. the zoster case mentioned at the beginning of this chapter), but usually the diagnostic process is hypothetico-deductive. We may teach medical students to take a full history and to do a complete physical examination, but the experienced clinician will soon generate diagnostic hypotheses which he then seeks to confirm or exclude by specific questions, by the physical examination and by paraclinical tests.

In this respect diagnostic thinking resembles scientific thinking as scientists engaged in innovative research will also generate hypotheses which they then subject to critical experiments. This analogy is interesting from the point of view that the mental process involved in the generation of scientific hypotheses is quite unknown and the same can be said about the generation of diagnostic hypotheses. The ability to make fruitful conjectures varies among scientists, and similar variation among doctors may help to explain that some are better diagnosticians than others. Obviously, theoretical knowledge and experience are also important as the clinician can only think of those diseases with which he is acquainted.

Diagnostic reasoning always includes probabilistic considerations. The initial diagnostic hypotheses, i.e. the tentative diagnoses, are all to a varying extent probable, and, gradually, the clinician must shorten the list of diagnostic possibilities. In complicated cases simple tests which provide reliable negative results may be used to eliminate some of the tentative diagnoses, and afterwards, when only few possibilities remain, more sophisticated tests which provide reliable positive results may be used to establish the final diagnosis.

The probabilistic considerations will rarely be exact, but there can be no doubt that the good diagnostician, even if he has never heard the expression, is an expert in Bayesian thinking. To explain that we shall once again look at Bayes' formula in its simple form. T + in this context may represent not only a positive test result, but also a particular clinical picture or a particular symptom or sign:

$$P(D+|T+) = P(T+|D+)\frac{P(D+)}{P(T+)}$$

The formula shows that in order to determine the probability of a particular diagnosis the clinician must be able to assess: (1) the probability of the clinical picture in question among patients with that disease, i.e. the nosographic TP probability or $P(T+|D+)$; (2) the probability that a patient in his practice has the disease (the practice prevalence), i.e. $P(D+)$; and (3) the probability that one of his patients presents that particular clinical picture, i.e. $P(T+)$.

The probability that an individual patient suffers from a particular disease, $P(D+|T+)$, is a subjective probability, but it is derived from the assessment of three frequential probabilities. Once again we are faced with the typical situation that a clinician uses his empirical knowledge about groups of patients to judge what is the matter with the individual patient.

The first of the three probabilities represents the clinician's nosographic knowledge, which he may have obtained by reading about the clinical presentation of the disease in the appropriate chapter of a medical textbook. When it is mentioned that a particular symptom, sign or clinical picture is very common, common or rare, those statements may be regarded as inexact noso-graphic TP probabilities. The two other probabilities are rarely recorded any-where and the clinician must rely on his uncontrolled experience.

As mentioned already the patients described in the textbooks may not cor-respond to those seen by the clinician, but nevertheless Bayesian thinking is required whenever textbook knowledge is used for diagnosing individual patients, and clinicians must be aware of the implications of this fact. It is, for instance, a common experience that newly fledged general practitioners tend to believe that their patients suffer from all sorts of rare diseases. They have had most of their training as junior hospital doctors and if, for instance, one of them has recently been employed at a gastroenterological hospital department he may well suspect that Crohn's disease is the most probable diagnosis in a patient with chronic diarrhoea. He is still programmed with the relatively high $P(D +)$ for that disease at the hospital and therefore he overestimates $P(D +| T +)$. Similar problems arise when a doctor trained in Europe moves, for instance, to Tanzania. He may have learnt his textbook on tropical diseases by heart, but he will not be a good diagnostician until he has also learnt to assess correctly the frequency of different diseases and the frequency of different clinical pictures in that part of the world.

Differences among clinicians as regards their ability to assess frequential probabilities and to convert them in the Bayesian way may well contribute to the variation in diagnostic skills.

This presentation might give the impression that the clinician's degree of confidence in a particular diagnosis, i.e. the subjective probability of the diag-nosis, is necessarily based on frequential considerations, but we have men-tioned already that this is not the case. The diagnostic strategy also includes deductive reasoning from theoretical knowledge. At the beginning of this chapter we mentioned the jaundiced patient where the consultant deduced from his knowledge about the excretion of bilirubin what might be wrong with the patient. In that case the list of tentative diagnoses was the result of deductive thinking. We may assume that the consultant proceeded by order-ing the appropriate blood tests and an ultrasound scan of the liver, and then by a combination of deductive and probabilistic reasoning reached the final diagnosis.

The choice of diagnostic strategy is further complicated by the fact that the clinician must take into account not only the probability that the patient suf-fers from different diseases, but also the consequences for the patient of mak-ing or not making a diagnosis. In some cases the consequences of missing a diagnosis are so grave that it must be excluded even in those cases where it is highly improbable. It may be considered necessary to do a lumbar puncture in a febrile patient to exclude an unlikely diagnosis of meningitis or to examine the colon of a patient with a fairly typical irritable bowel syndrome in order to exclude that the symptoms are caused by a colonic cancer.

In other cases the probability of a disease may be rather high, but it may still not be justified to pursue that diagnosis. This would be the case if a chest X-ray reveals a shadow in the lung which might well be caused by a cancer, if the patient's clinical condition prohibits further action. There seems to be a tendency in contemporary hospital practice to subject old patients to too many diagnostic investigations of no consequence.

The clinician must also take into account other consequences of his decisions. Some diagnostic procedures are unpleasant for the patient and may even be associated with a small risk of complications, and others are expensive. Economical considerations are, of course, particularly important in a national health service with a fixed budget (Chapter 7).

Diagnostic strategy is often a balancing act. The clinician must not overlook diseases in need of treatment and he must not make a diagnosis when it is not warranted. Meador once reported a particularly crude example of 'over-diagnosis' [94,95] or, to use his own expression, the tendency to make a diagnosis of 'nondisease' which is then used to justify a therapeutic decision. In the 1930s, 1000 school children in New York were seen sequentially by four different groups of doctors who were unaware of the fact that the children had been seen or would be seen by other doctors. The first group of doctors found that 611 of the 1000 children had undergone tonsillectomy or were in need of that operation. The second group of doctors saw the remaining 389 children and judged that 174 of them were in need of tonsillectomy, and then the residual 215 children were seen by the third group of doctors who advised tonsillectomy on an additional 99. The last 116 children were seen by the fourth group who suggested tonsillectomy in 65. Now only 51 of the 1000 children were left. Tonsillectomy for 'chronic tonsillitis' is still sometimes done.

There are other historical examples of nondisease, such as the diagnosis of gastroptosis, an elongated colon or chronic appendicitis, and possibly the recent diagnosis 'chronic fatigue syndrome' belongs to the same category. This is a controversial issue, and we do not deny that some virus infections are followed by a prolonged period of fatigue, but in many cases the justification of this diagnostic label seems doubtful. Patients with psychosocial problems often receive unwarranted somatic diagnoses although, usually, they are less fanciful than this new syndrome.

Chapter 4

The inherent complexity of diagnostic reasoning explains that the diagnostic process cannot be reduced to a simple algorithm and it was only to be expected that, so far, computer diagnosis has not been much of a success. It also explains that diagnostic skills cannot be learnt from textbooks alone, but also require bedside teaching.

CHAPTER 5

Uncontrolled Experience

Errare humanum est sed in errore perseverare turpe
(To err is human but to repeat the error is shameful). [Old saying]

Treatment may take many forms, from advice about change of life style to drug therapy and surgery, and the objects of therapeutic decisions are equally varied. We use such terms as symptomatic, causal, curative, palliative and prophylactic treatment, and clinicians must always bear in mind what effect they wish to obtain by a given therapeutic measure. In bronchial asthma, for instance, they may treat patients with bronchodilating agents or cortico-steroids either to stop the acute attack or to prevent new attacks, and they may treat cancer patients with chemotherapy either to cure or to palliate.

Clinicians must also consider why they expect a treatment to have the desired effect, and here there are three possibilities:

1   Deduction from theory. Theoretical knowledge of disease mechanisms and the mechanism of action of the treatment in question makes the clinician believe that the treatment is effective.

2   Uncontrolled experience. The clinician herself and other clinicians are convinced, by their everyday experience, that the treatment is effective.

3   Controlled experience. Well-controlled clinical research, preferably in the form of randomized clinical trials, has provided convincing evidence that the treatment is effective.

We are, of course, on very firm ground if we know how the treatment works, if there is a consensus of opinion that it does work, and if randomized clinical trials have given the expected results, but unfortunately this ideal requirement is rarely fulfilled. Therefore, it is necessary to discuss separately the three possible reasons for expecting a therapeutic response, and in this connection we should not forget the lesson of medical history.

Uncontrolled experience in a pre-scientific era

There are many examples that the uncontrolled experience of both medical doctors and lay people have made important contributions to clinical medicine, and we shall mention a few of these.

The story of scurvy is a good example of the inertia of medical progress in former days [19,23,96]. The toll of this disease was extremely heavy when the Europeans began to explore the world across the oceans; on some of the longest sea voyages the majority of the seamen died. The Spaniards and the Dutch had noted the effect of lemons as early as the sixteenth century and so did Richard Hawkins and James Lancaster in about 1600, but for a long time this uncontrolled experience did not gain general recognition. In 1747 James Lind did an experiment where 12 patients with scurvy received different treatments; only two of these, who were given lemons and oranges, improved. Lind himself was not convinced, but the same year John Huxham reported that, in contrast to ordinary seamen, officers who carried wine, cider, lemons and fresh provisions did not get scurvy. He also described how the disease was cured when the seamen reached harbour and got 'proper food and herbage' [97]. Finally, in 1795 the Admiralty ordered the issue of lemon juice in the Royal Navy.

Popular medicine has also provided effective treatments. In the eighteenth century an old woman in Shropshire observed that a drug containing more than 20 different herbs had a beneficial effect on dropsy [62], and the general practitioner, William Withering, found that the active component was fox-glove (*Digitalis purpurea*). In 1785 he described the effect in a number of cases, including this one: 'A man about 50 years of age . . . complained to me of an asthma . . . His breath was very short, his countenance was sunken, his belly large; and upon examination a fluctuation in it was very perceptible. His urine for some time past had been small in quantity. I directed a decoction of Fo. Digital. recent. which made him very sick, the sickness occurring at intervals for several days, during which time he made a large quantity of water. His breath gradually drew easier, his belly subsided, and in about 10 days he begun to eat with a keen appetite' [98].

The introduction of vaccination against smallpox has an important place in the history of prophylaxis. It was prompted by the experience that people who had had cowpox were spared during smallpox epidemics. Jenner, who in 1798 had practised vaccination for some years, applied for permission to present his results to the Royal Society in London. This request was refused, because 'he ought not to risk his reputation by presenting to the learned body anything which appeared so much at variance with established knowledge and withal so incredible' [20]. However, as it often happens in the history of medicine, 'the established knowledge' was disproved, and this new preventive treatment soon received widespread acceptance.

These examples illustrate that the uncontrolled experience of doctors and laymen have made important contributions to clinical practice, and they also inspired theoretical research. Vaccination against smallpox became the fore-runner of immunization against many infectious diseases, and the treatment of scurvy ultimately led to the discovery of vitamins. We usually talk of basic research in the laboratory and applied research at the bedside, but often the situation is reversed.

These examples may well give the impression that the history of medicine is a success story, but we must not forget the seamy side of clinical practice in former days. It was realized even at the time of Hippocrates that clinical experi-ence may be fallacious (*experientia fallax est*), and there seems to be no limit to the number of absurd and sometimes harmful treatments which doctors have used in the course of time.

The Frenchman Amboise Paré, who for a time was a military surgeon, fol-lowed the usual routine of treating gunshot wounds by cauterization with boiling oil. However, during a campaign in Italy in 1536, he ran out of oil and instead he had to apply some indifferent concoction. He lay sleepless all night fearing the fate of the unfortunate soldiers who had been treated so uncon-ventionally, and he was much surprised the next morning when he found these soldiers 'free from vehemencie of paine to have had good rest', whereas those soldiers who had been treated correctly were feverish and tormented with pain. Until then numerous soldiers had been exposed to the barbarity of caut-erization with a hot iron or with boiling oil. One of the less edifying of Hip-pocrates' aphorisms runs as follows: 'What medicine does not cure is cured by the knife, what the knife does not cure, is cured by the iron, and what the iron does not cure must be considered incurable' [21,99].

Enemata were already popular in ancient Egypt, and according to Pliny the enema originated from the observation that the ibis used its curved beak to give itself rectal infusions of Nile water [21]. Since then a variety of rectal infu-sions have been used in a variety of diseases. In the seventeenth century, rectal infusion of wine was used against consumption, urine enemata were used against dropsy, and holy water enemata were used to exorcize devils from pos-sessed nuns. In the eighteenth century tobacco-smoke clysters were recom-mended for the resuscitation of drowned persons.

Blood-letting and leeching is a chapter in itself. From classical antiquity to the nineteenth century, blood-letting performed in a variety of ways was a standard treatment of almost any disease. Broussais (1772–1838), who was a highly esteemed professor of pathology in Paris, has been called the most sanguinary physician in history [21]. During the cholera epidemic in 1832 he advocated that the patients were treated with a strict diet and blood-letting by phlebotomy and leeching. A strict diet meant that the patients were not allowed to eat or drink. It has been calculated that 85 000 L of blood were let at Parisian hospitals in the year 1800 [6]; in 1824 France imported 33 million leeches [62] and the British Isles bought 5 million [21]. Leeches have been used far into the twentieth century.

The perusal of any old textbook of medicine reveals page after page of meaningless treatments. Of course, we cannot know with certainty whether some of the herbs had pharmacological effects which are unknown to us, but by and large we must presume that medical treatment with few exceptions, such as the use of opiates, was quite useless until the end of the nineteenth century. One cannot imagine, for example, that any beneficial effect was obtained by the treatment of a mad dog's bite with angelica root [30], diabetes or pisspot disease with burnt hedgehog (eighteenth-century England) or gastric ulcer with cantharides (nineteenth-century Denmark) [79].

The numerical method

At the beginning of the nineteenth century all treatment was still based on speculative theories about the causes of disease and uncontrolled experience, but scientific thinking slowly gained ground. The foundation of modern statistics had been laid, and in the 1830s the first attempts were made to apply statistical methods to clinical medicine. This happened in Paris, and Gavaret's book from 1840 about the principles for the use of statistics in medicine [100] is still very exciting reading. He introduced the concept of confidence intervals, and in 10 tenets he warned clinicians against drawing conclusions from therapeutic experience based on small numbers of patients. The sixth tenet states: 'in order to prefer one therapeutic method to another, the results must not only be better, but the difference must exceed a certain limit which depends on the number of the collected cases'. This book, which includes tables for the calculation of confidence intervals, is more than a hundred years ahead of its time. Gavaret's novel ideas spread to other countries in Europe, and in Denmark, for instance, they had some impact. A young Danish doctor, C.E. Fenger, who later became Minister of Finance, had heard Gavaret's lectures in Paris, and on his return in 1839 he wrote two papers on the numerical method in the newly started *Danish Medical Journal* [101]. He was depressed by the state of contemporary clinical medicine and believed that greater stringency could only be achieved by the introduction of statistical methods. He used pneumonia as an example, and made a critical analysis of diagnosis, prognosis and treatment in numerical terms. He calculated conditional probabilities and stressed that prognostic studies must be related to the clinical pattern. However, the idea that progress in clinical medicine is dependent on observations made with 'order and care on a sufficient number of exactly recorded cases' was too revolutionary for some contemporary colleagues. A regimental surgeon rushed into print with a letter to the editor. The numerical method, he wrote, contains something good and something new. 'What a shame that the good is not new and that the new is not good'. He asserted that the numerical method lets quantity outweigh quality; it ignores the individuality of patients and underrates the experience of skilled clinicians. Similar arguments are still heard nowadays from those who are opposed to evidence-based medicine.

That debate in France and abroad started a development which in the long run proved to be self-effacing. P.C.A. Louis had for a number of years studied the prognosis of patients with acute infectious diseases who were bled either earlier or later during the course of their disease. He found that the prognosis did not depend on the time of the phlebotomy and concluded in his book, published in 1835, that blood-letting had only small influence on the course of pneumonia, erysipelas and diphtheria [102]. He did not perform controlled therapeutic trials, but his observations were felt to be convincing and created great uneasiness in the medical world. The dogma that patients with acute infections had to be bled as quickly as possible had been universally accepted, and now Louis cast doubt on this mainstay of therapy. One might have expected that the adherents of the numerical school would have begun to test critically all those treatments which they used, but that did not happen. Instead, they simply lost faith in their therapeutic remedies, and clinical medicine entered a period which has aptly been labelled therapeutic nihilism. Louis had won a victory, but it was dearly bought. What was lost was not only a number of useless or harmful treatments, but clinicians' interest in clinical research [61].

Towards the end of the century a revival of critical clinical thinking was seen in Poland, and Bieganski discussed many of those topics which are also considered in this book, but this interesting intermezzo in the history of medicine was short-lived and had little international impact [103,104].

The biostatistical approach to clinical medicine which had been introduced by Louis and Gavaret was almost forgotten for more than a century.

The era of laboratory research

The new development which originated in this vacuum proved more viable. Scientifically minded doctors realized that the time-honoured speculative disease theories had to be rejected, and that they would not be able to develop rational treatments unless they gained new knowledge about the pathogenesis of different diseases. Intellectually, they turned their backs to the everyday problems of clinical practice and retired to the newly established research laboratories.

Myxoedema was one of those diseases which attracted the interest of the medical scientists. It had been described as a disease entity in the 1870s, and a few years later Kocher and Reverdin from Switzerland observed the same clinical picture after thyroidectomy. In 1884 Schiff found that experimental myxoedema in dogs could be prevented by a previous thyroid graft, and this finding led Murray to treat myxoedema with injections of thyroid extract. Howitz of Copenhagen introduced oral treatment in 1892 and myxoedema became the first disease to be fully controlled by pharmacotherapy. The example illustrates the interplay between clinical and laboratory research on an international scale which continues today. The later development need not be discussed in detail. The introduction of insulin treatment of diabetes, treatment of pernicious anaemia with raw liver and later vitamin B_{12}, and treatment of infectious diseases with sulphonamides and penicillin are well-known milestones.

However, as Lasègue (1810–83) said about his laboratory-orientated colleagues [18], 'They explain much or rather they explain everything and they pass quickly from hypothesis to practice'. Doctors have always had a tendency to overestimate their theoretical knowledge and that may easily lead to the introduction of ineffective or harmful treatments. They believe that they fully understand the pathogenesis of a disease and the mechanism of action of some treatment, but unfortunately the human organism is so complex that it is rarely possible to predict with certainty the effect of a new treatment. Only experience can show whether a treatment is more beneficial than harmful, and as long as that experience was uncontrolled, the situation remained much the same as in the pre-scientific era.

Anticoagulant treatment of myocardial infarction is a good example. In the 1950s the coagulation mechanisms of the blood attracted considerable interest. The disease myocardial infarction was in those days called coronary thrombosis and it was considered rational to treat the patients with the newly discovered vitamin K antagonists. Papers were published where clinicians reported their excellent results and soon the treatment was accepted on both sides of the Atlantic. At that time randomized clinical trials (as described in Chapter 6) were still very rare, but when they were done 10 years later it was found that the treatment with vitamin K antagonists had no beneficial effect in this disease.

Oxygen treatment of chronic respiratory failure also illustrates that apparently rational treatments may be dangerous. Anybody with a little knowledge of respiratory physiology will realize that cyanosed and dyspnoeic patients suffer from hypoxia, but treatment with oxygen at high concentrations must have caused the death of thousands of patients until the danger of carbon dioxide narcosis was realized in the 1950s. At that time it was not possible to monitor the carbon dioxide concentration of arterial blood and it was only too easy to misinterpret the course of the clinical events. Imagine a cyanosed patient who is given too much oxygen. His colour improves almost immediately, his respiration is 'normalized', he falls asleep due to exhaustion and later he dies 'in spite of' the treatment.

The treatment of duodenal ulcer shows to which extent a generation of gastroenterologists were misled by uncontrolled experience. In the 1960s most patients were given a bland diet, an anticholinergic and an antacid whenever needed to relieve pain. Diet was the first of the treatments to be proved worthless, and in 1970 a carefully designed therapeutic trial showed that two commonly used anticholinergics had no appreciable clinical effect [105]; in a leading article in the *Lancet* they were aptly called 'logical placebos' [106]. Few clinicians, however, doubted the specific effect of antacids on ulcer pain, and it came as a surprise when it was found some years later that a placebo preparation relieved the pain just as well as a potent liquid antacid [107]. Then, for a time, no treatments were believed to be effective, until a new randomized trial showed that intensive antacid therapy, contrary to expectations, greatly enhanced ulcer healing [108]. Since then, of course, the introduction of new, effective treatments has changed the picture.

Today we still use treatments which have not been adequately tested, and undoubtedly future generations of doctors will realize that some of them are totally useless. There is no reason to believe that our aptitude for drawing the right conclusions from clinical practice is any better than that of our predecessors. However, it remains to answer the question why clinicians throughout the history of medicine have been fooled by their uncontrolled experience, and in order to do so it is necessary to consider five different factors: ignorance of the spontaneous course of the disease; imprecision of clinical data and regression towards the mean; runs of good or bad luck; psychological and other kinds of bias; and the placebo effect.

The spontaneous course of the disease

Treatment of different diseases has at all times to a large extent been stand-ardized, and doctors who always treat patients with the same disease in the same manner are bound to lose touch with the course of the disease when no treatment is given. Therefore, it is only to be expected that doctors, when treating diseases of short duration, sometimes mistake spontaneous recovery for an effect of their therapeutic efforts. In 1809, for instance, a doctor recom-mended belladonna as a remedy against whooping cough as 'the cough disap-pears after 6 or 8 weeks, occasionally earlier' [109]. Probably, this observation was correct but it should not be attributed to the treatment. Admittedly, it is easy in the daily routine to interpret simple coincidence as a causal relation-ship. When urinary tract infections are treated with sulphonamide and the symptoms subside within a few days, it is tempting to conclude that the treat-ment was effective, but once in a while it is revealed that this was not the case. That happens when in due time the result of the urine culture arrives and it is disclosed that the bacteria were resistant to sulphonamide.

Similar misinterpretations find their way to the medical journals. In 1994 readers of reviews in the *British Medical Journal* [110] and the *Lancet* [111] were informed that it was possible, using certain treatments, to stop bleeding in 90–95% of patients with bleeding oesophageal varices. That suggests a huge treatment effect, but the authors failed to mention that the rate of spon-taneous bleeding arrest is very high in the control groups of randomized trials.

It may also be difficult to judge correctly a treatment effect in chronic diseases. The severity of the symptoms in ulcerative colitis, bronchial asthma, rheumatoid arthritis and numerous other conditions fluctuate, as illustrated by Fig. 16

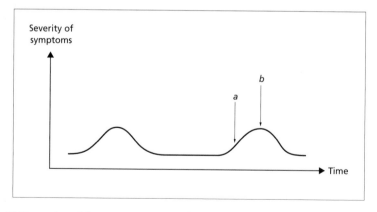

Fig. 16 Fluctuations of disease activity in a case of ulcerative colitis. See text for further explanation.

and clinicians may easily be deceived if they ignore this fact. Imagine a patient with ulcerative colitis who has been symptom-free for a long period of time and then suffers a relapse. After a while (at point *a* on the curve) she decides to see a doctor, who then refers her to a specialist. The severity of the symptoms continues to increase until the specialist finds time to see her (at point *b* on the curve), but at that time she is on the verge of a spontaneous remission and any treatment will appear to be effective. Naturally, this course of events is by no means a certainty, but it may happen sufficiently often to make the specialist inform her colleagues that, according to her personal experience, the treatment used helps a considerable number of patients with ulcerative colitis.

Another example illustrates the same phenomenon particularly well. It was once believed that X-ray treatment was effective in osteoarthritis and spondylosis, and the patients were told that sometimes the effect would show immediately, sometimes it would only be evident after a few weeks, and sometimes the pain would get worse before the effect set in. This experience was probably quite right apart from the fact that it was the spontaneous fluctuations of the disease and not the treatment effect which was described. We should remember that patients tend to seek our advice when their symptoms are getting worse.

Imprecision of clinical data and regression towards the mean

On page 36 we introduced the concept of regression towards the mean. If we determine the serum cholesterol in a number of patients whose cholesterol level is completely normal, then we must expect, due to the imprecision (limited reproducibility) of the chemical analysis, that some of the results are high and others low. If we repeat the measurements some days later (still assuming that the patients' cholesterol levels are normal) we shall also obtain some high results and some low results, but probably not in the same patients. The cholesterol will seem to fall if initially it was high, and rise if it was low. This regularity is to be expected whenever we repeat the observation of a variable phenomenon twice. If we observe the flow of traffic, we shall probably find that a very large car is followed by a smaller car, and that a very small car is followed by a larger car. Galton reported in 1885 that tall parents usually had children who were shorter than themselves, whereas short parents usually had taller children [112].

Regression towards the mean may simulate a treatment effect. If, for instance, the serum cholesterol is measured once in all patients with ischaemic heart disease, and treatment is instituted in all those with a high value, a decrease in the serum cholesterol will be recorded at the next visit in a number of cases, whether or not the treatment had any effect. That is to be expected due to the analytic imprecision, but the phenomenon is further accentuated by the day-to-day variation of the patients' cholesterol levels. The same applies to blood pressure measurements where day-to-day variation may be caused both by the imprecision of the recording of the blood pressure and by fluctuations of the actual blood pressure. No doubt some patients are treated unnecessarily for years because their doctor only measured their blood pressure once before treatment was instituted.

The apparent improvement of chronically ill patients with a fluctuating course, as described above, is one more example of regression towards the mean, due to the fact that clinicians usually see their patients when the symptoms are at their worst.

The interpretation of descriptive data may also be confounded by regression towards the mean if the reproducibility is not perfect, i.e. if kappa in inter- or intra-observer studies is less than 1. If, for instance, a series of patients with ulcer symptoms are subjected to a duodenoscopy twice, the diagnoses may well differ, as it is possible to miss the ulcer and as the distinction between an erosion and a small ulcer is somewhat subjective. Sometimes an ulcer will be diagnosed the first time, but not the second time, and sometimes an ulcer will not be diagnosed the first time, but only the second time. Imagine then that a gastroenterologist treats only those patients with ulcer symptoms who are found to have an ulcer and subjects these to a repeat duodenoscopy a few weeks later. Even if no ulcers have healed, she will record that the ulcer has 'disappeared' in some patients and she may interpret this finding as a treatment effect. This is a common phenomenon. If the second assessment of the pulmonary scintigrams in the example in Chapter 2 (p. 26) had represented the assessment of a new set of scans after treatment for one month, one might have concluded that the cure rate was about 50% as the number of positive scintigrams had fallen from 22 to 11. The phenomenon is also bound to occur in some randomized clinical trials, where it may explain some of the 'cures' in untreated control groups.

Run of luck

Clinicians' personal experience is often limited to a relatively small number of cases and they may easily be deceived by a run of good or bad luck. It is encouraging if 40 (or 80%) out of 50 patients are cured by a new surgical operation, especially if the prognosis without surgery is known to be very poor, but it is necessary to ask the question to what extent such limited experience is reliable.

This is a statistical problem which may be illustrated by a simple model. We may imagine a chest of drawers filled with a very large number of black and white marbles. These marbles symbolize all present and future patients with the disease in question, i.e. the hypothetical population of patients. The white marbles represent those patients who are cured by the operation, whereas the black marbles represent those who die. The percentage of white and black marbles in the chest is unknown.

From this chest we sample 50 marbles at random, and we find that 40 are white and 10 are black. Then the question is asked: What can we conclude from this sample as regards the true percentage of white marbles in the chest?

Common sense tells us that the true percentage of white marbles could be, say, 78% or 81%, since the slightly different percentage in our small sample may easily be attributed to chance. Common sense also tells us that it is very unlikely that the true percentage is, say, 10% or 15%, because we do not expect chance to cheat us that much. Somebody who is well versed in statistical calculations can handle this problem in exact numerical terms, since she can calculate the probability of obtaining our result given any percentage of white marbles in the chest, and by means of such calculations she can tell us within what limits the true percentage may be expected to lie. In this case she will inform us, using the conventional statistical terminology, that the lower and upper 95% confidence limits are 66.3% and 90.0%, or in other words the 95% confidence interval is 66.3% to 90.0%.

It is easiest to explain the concept of confidence intervals by making a distinction between rare and common events and by defining rare events as those that occur less than 5% of times. Using this definition, the calculation has shown that the observed cure rate of 80% would have been a rare event if the true cure rate was lower than the lower confidence limit or larger than the upper confidence limit. When we calculate the 95% confidence interval we shall, in the long run, be right 19 out of 20 times when we make the assumption that the interval includes the true value.

It does not follow from this argument, however, that we should feel 95% confident that the confidence interval in a particular study includes the true value. Imagine, for instance, that we do a thorough search of the literature that reveals that other surgeons who did the same operation on average only cured 60% of their patients. Then we must seriously consider the possibility that the results obtained by this surgeon only represented a run of good luck. In other

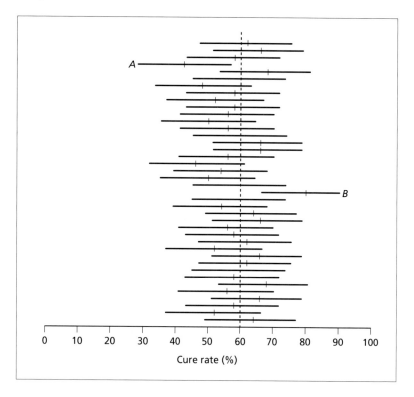

Fig. 17 Forty equally-skilled surgeons carry out the same operation on a series of 50 patients. It is assumed that the true cure rate is 60%. The figure shows the observed cure rate (with 95% confidence interval) for each series.

words, we should no longer be almost sure, i.e. 95% confident, that the true cure rate fell within the interval. We should have to consider the possibility that her result was one of the rare events where the true value falls outside the interval.

Figure 17 illustrates the expected variation of the results, if the true cure rate were exactly 60%, and if 40 equally proficient surgeons, independently of one another, had done a series of 50 operations on similar patients. The observed cure rate and the 95% confidence interval are shown for each of these series, and it is seen that in most cases the interval includes the true cure rate of 60%. In one series (*A*), however, the true cure rate exceeds the upper confidence limit, and in another (*B*) it is lower than the lower confidence limit.

If the true cure rate was, in fact, 60%, our surgeon's result would correspond to the series marked *B*, but we cannot exclude the alternative explanation that she is, in fact, more skilled than her colleagues and that the true cure rate in her case is higher. To prove that she would have to do the operation on many more patients.

The distinction between frequential (statistical) and subjective probabilities, which was introduced in Chapter 4 (p. 87), is important in this context. Statisticians concern themselves with frequential probabilities; they tell us that in the long run we shall be right 19 out of 20 times when we make the assumption that the true value falls within the 95% confidence interval. Readers of medical journals, on the other hand, wish to assess the subjective probability of (their confidence in) the assumption that the interval includes the true value in a particular study, and that assessment is based not only on the results of that study, but also on other kinds of information, such as the results of other studies or, in this case, additional information about the surgeon. We should, for instance, feel more confident that she is doing better than her colleagues, if she also has a reputation of being more deft than others when she does other types of surgical operations. Therefore, the expression 95% confidence interval is a misnomer. It reflects the statistical way of thinking and does not tell us how confident we should be in the individual case.

It follows that confidence intervals must always be interpreted with care, but nonetheless they are of fundamental importance in the context of evidence-based medicine, both when we assess our own clinical experience critically and when we assess the results of others from articles in medical journals. The exact figures reported in the journals only refer to those patients who were observed by the author, and the paper has little scientific relevance unless we assess to what extent those results can be extrapolated to other patients, especially our own. The determination of confidence intervals serves this important purpose.

The calculation of the exact interval (from the binomial distribution) is a laborious, iterative process, but that problem is bypassed by the use of statistical tables [113] and computer programs. It will be found that the width of the confidence interval depends on the number of patients, which is only to be expected as greater experience allows more precise predictions. If the surgeon had observed that 8 of 10 patients were cured, the interval would have been 44.4% to 97.5%, and, if she had observed that 80 out of 100 were cured, the interval would have been 70.8% to 87.3%.

It is also possible to make rough estimates of the width of confidence intervals by doing a bit of mental arithmetic, and the following formula (where N is number of patients) may be used for that purpose: 95% confidence interval = observed cure rate ± $100/\sqrt{N}$. If, for instance, we have observed that 50 of 100 patients are cured, the confidence interval is 40%–60%. If we have found that 200 of 400 patients are cured, the interval is 45%–55%. This calculation, however, is only valid when the observed rate does not differ too much from 50%, as the interval gradually becomes narrower and more asymmetric when the observed rate approaches 0% or 100%. When 40 of 50 patients are cured the 95% confidence interval is not 76%–94% (as one would expect from the formula), but, as we have seen, 66%–90%.

Bias

A distinction must be made between random variation and bias (systematic errors) (p. 20). Regression towards the mean and runs of bad or good luck illustrate the influence of random variation, but uncontrolled clinical experience may also be distorted by different kinds of bias.

Previously, clinicians often published the results they had obtained by treating a series of patients, but the scientific value of such studies was very small. Usually, the diagnostic criteria, the indications for using the treatment and the criteria for assessing the effects, were not defined in advance, and in that case there are numerous sources of bias. Possibly, the severely ill (or mildly ill) patients were not included, and possibly, the final diagnosis which determined the inclusion in the series was influenced by the treatment result. In general, little attention should be paid to studies which are not prospective and which have not been carried out according to a detailed protocol.

Even well planned studies of the effect of some treatment are of little use if there is no control group, except perhaps in the context of quality assurance. If, for example, the outcome of a particular surgical operation varies at different surgical departments, one should, of course, explore the possible reasons for that variation.

The reliability of uncontrolled series of treatment results is particularly low if the results have been recorded nowhere but in the memory of the physician, as those cases which took an unusual course stick to the mind much more easily than the others. If we ask a colleague to tell us about the effect of a particular treatment, she will be inclined to overestimate the benefits if some patients fared surprisingly well, and she may warn us against the treatment, if a few patients fared surprisingly badly. This phenomenon is called *recall bias*, and the exceptional cases may very well have an undue influence on the treatment of future patients. Once a single case of cerebral haemorrhage due to anticoagulant treatment made a clinician refrain from using that treatment even when it was clearly indicated.

Psychological bias is also important. Clinicians hope that their patients get better and that their treatments are successful. That is of course a laudable attitude, but it also has the effect that clinicians are biased observers. They convince themselves that the patients look a little better or that the symptoms are a little less severe. This optimism may create a psychological game between doctor and patient with the result that the patient, too, says that she feels a little better either because she believes so or because she wishes to please the doctor.

The placebo effect

The word placebo means 'I shall please' and it was first used in the context of medical treatment towards the end of the 18th century. In *Motherby's New Medical Dictionary* from 1785 placebo is defined as 'a commonplace method or medicine calculated to amuse for a time, rather than for any other purpose' [11].

Since then expressions like placebo, placebo phenomena, placebo treatment and placebo effect have gained access both within and without the medical profession, also when no allusion is made to the therapist's intentions, and confusion reigns. Much has been written about this topic, but no generally accepted stringent definition exists [114–117].

We hope, however, that we capture the essence of the usual meaning of the expression when we define a placebo effect as the therapeutic effect of the treatment setting as a whole, including the doctor–patient relationship, i.e. a beneficial effect which cannot be explained by direct interference with physiological and metabolic processes. The alleged effect may be increased well-being, alleviation of specific symptoms (typically pain), normalization of objective findings or the prevention of disease or disease complications. One may also talk about a 'negative' placebo effect or a nocebo effect (derived from latin *nocere* = harm), if the patient's condition gets worse.

Clinicians often report that they observed a beneficial effect of the prescription of a drug, which they themselves regarded as completely ineffective. If the drug was given as tablets, they may even use the term 'placebo tablets', but taken literally that is misleading, as it is not implied that the tablets themselves had a mysterious effect. It is the prescription of the tablets which is believed to be effective, and it is not suggested that they would have had a similar effect, if, for instance, they had been given to a laboratory animal or if the patient had found them in the street. It is also believed that the placebo phenomenon may play an important role when clinicians prescribe drugs with a well-established specific effect (e.g. antirheumatic drugs which inhibit the synthesis of prostaglandins in both humans and animals), as the observed treatment result may then be regarded as the sum of the specific effect and a placebo effect.

The analysis of the placebo concept raises two kinds of questions, firstly ontological questions, i.e. questions about the true nature of the phenomenon, and empirical questions, i.e. questions concerning the demonstration of the phenomenon by means of clinical research.

Even those who take the placebo effect for granted have rarely thought much about its true nature, but it is usually assumed that it is a purely psychological or psychosomatic mechanism. It is not the treatment itself, but the patient's subjective experience of the setting in which the treatment takes place that elicits the response. The concept of psychosomatic mechanisms is disputed by some, but medical doctors accept that the sensation of fear may cause adrenalin release, a rise in blood pressure and palpitations, and if only we accept that, it is not such a mysterious idea that other subjective experiences may have a beneficial effect. Psychosomatic theory is related to those philosophical body–mind theories, according to which mental phenomena such as anxiety, hunger, pain and even negative and positive expectations may cause bodily phenomena. Some philosophers, e.g. behaviourists, would dispute that, but their theories seem incompatible with the subjective experience of most people [25].

It has been asserted that some phenomena which are usually regarded as placebo effects can be explained within conventional physiological theory. Some patients are reported to respond similarly to an active analgesic and to an inactive preparation, as regards the onset and the cessation of pain relief, and this effect might be caused by a conditioned reflex which was established during previous treatment with analgesics. Pain relief is also reported after the injection of saline or acupuncture, and it has been suggested that the effect in those cases is caused by the release of endorphins. However, a critical review of the relevant studies concluded that none of these hypotheses have been convincingly documented [118]. If the explanations were true, it would have been disproved that the effects in question were placebo effects, at least according to our definition.

These speculations about the true nature of the placebo phenomenon do not tell us how to demonstrate and perhaps measure placebo effects. Most of the studies which are quoted again and again by those who emphasize the great significance of the placebo phenomenon are simply observations on series of patients who received a treatment which was considered pharmacologically inactive. It is, for instance, often mentioned that 'placebo treatment' relieves headache in about 80% of cases. The observation is probably correct, but the spontaneous course of an attack of headache was not taken into account. This kind of report made Beecher conclude in a much quoted paper that in various conditions the placebo effect is on average 35% [119].

The introduction of the randomized clinical trial stimulated the interest in the placebo phenomenon, which was then regarded as a source of error that might confound the interpretation of the results. Double-blind studies were recommended where the patients in the control group received inactive tablets, e.g. lactose tablets. Unfortunately, these tablets are often called placebo tablets, just as the control group is called the placebo group, and the effect observed in the control group is called the placebo effect. Using this terminology, the placebo effect in duodenal ulcer trials may be said to vary between 30% and 60%, as the healing rates in the control groups are of this order of magnitude. It cannot of course be excluded that the patients' expectations may promote ulcer healing, but the observed effect among the controls is also easily explained by a combination of spontaneous healing and, as explained above, regression towards the mean due to observer variation.

The assessment of the placebo effect requires trials that are especially designed for that purpose. One may, for instance, do randomized trials with three groups of patients, one of which receives pharmacologically active treatment, another 'placebo treatment' (pharmacologically inactive tablets) and a third 'no treatment', but even this design does not solve the problem as 'no treatment' is part of a clinical setting which may be associated with either a positive or negative placebo effect. One may also do trials with two groups of patients, where the alleged placebo stimulus is maximized in one group and minimized in the other. The patients in one group may be offered lengthy consultations while those in the other are just kept on the waiting list [114]. A variety of designs have been used, but unfortunately many of the studies have methodological flaws. A Dutch group that reviewed hundreds of articles only recovered four which they thought were acceptable [120].

At present it is very difficult to distinguish between what we believe and what we really know about the placebo phenomenon, and systematic reviews of the placebo literature, including meta-analyses of randomized trials, are greatly needed. The Cochrane Collaboration (see p. 140) is active in the field, and it is hoped that their efforts will help to clarify the issues. Here only a few studies will be mentioned.

One randomized trial suggests that the physician's attitude and the information given to the patient are of considerable importance [121]. A general practitioner did a trial where 200 patients with non-specific symptoms, i.e. symptoms which were not explained by a particular diagnosis, were allocated at random to four groups: positive or negative consultations with or without treatment. At the positive consultations the patients received a 'fake diagnosis' and were informed that they would soon feel much better. They were either told that no treatment was needed, or they were given inactive tablets with the information that they would have a good effect. At the negative consultations the clinician told the patients that he did not know what was wrong and that therefore he could prescribe no treatment, or he prescribed inactive tablets with the additional information that it was not certain that they would have any effect. Improvement was recorded in 64 of those 100 patients who received a positive consultation, and only in 39 of 100 patients who received a negative consultation; the prescription of inactive tablets seemed to make no difference. This trial, of course, presents considerable ethical and methodological problems, but we shall not discuss these.

Such trials and everyday experience suggest that the clinician's attitude, her confidence in the prescribed treatment and the information given to the patients may influence the way in which they perceive their symptoms and their general condition. Under those circumstances the technical term, a placebo effect, seems somewhat unnecessary. It is only to be expected that patients who worry about some subjective symptom will feel relieved when they hear that it is not serious. This was true of a colleague who once developed pain in the chest irradiating to the left arm; he was naturally worried, but when the typical vesicular eruption of herpes zoster appeared, the pain bothered him no longer.

Other randomized trials show more tangible effects of the clinical setting. It has, for instance, been reported that the presence of a person providing continuous support to women during childbirth had the following effects: the rates of caesarian sections, anaesthesia, analgesics and episiotomy were lower than among those women who received ordinary hospital care; further, the child was in a better condition at birth and there were fewer cases of severe postpartum depression [122]. It is not easy to interpret these results, but it cannot be excluded that the feeling of security induced by the continuous presence of another person had a beneficial psychosomatic effect. Objective placebo effects, e.g. improved healing of peptic ulcers, have also been reported in some studies, but these observations are not well documented.

It is sometimes argued by clinicians who give great credence to the placebo phenomenon that it may be justified to prescribe inactive treatments and to suggest to the patient, either implicitly or explicitly, that the treatment is effective. This practice is quite unacceptable from an ethical point of view, as it is hard to conceive that any patient seeking medical assistance expects to be wilfully deceived. However, recognition of the placebo concept may induce clinicians to pay greater attention to the human aspects of the doctor–patient relationship. It is very likely that a clinician who shows a genuine interest in the patient's situation and takes the necessary time to explain the results of investigations and the nature of the patient's disease will induce a greater placebo effect than the colleague who prescribes inactive tablets.

The need for controlled experience

Uncontrolled experience cannot be trusted and therefore it is necessary to test new treatments by means of controlled trials, i.e. trials where the effect of the new treatment is compared with the effect of the standard treatment or no treatment at all. This can be done in a number of ways.

One may simply introduce the new treatment in the daily routine and record the treatment result in a series of patients. Then these results are compared with those which were obtained in a series of historical controls, i.e. patients who during a preceding period received the old treatment. This procedure, however, cannot be recommended. Usually, the historical data are retrieved from the patients' notes, which are rarely sufficiently reliable to serve scientific purposes, but there are other sources of error. The adjuvant treatment may have been improved from the first period to the next, or the diagnostic methods may have been refined with the result that those patients who received the new treatment were less severely ill than those who received the old treatment. That was probably one of the reasons why the introduction of anticoagulant therapy in the 1950s was accompanied by a fall in the fatality rate of myocardial infarction (p. 98). Studies of this kind will also be biased if the clinicians refrain from treating severely ill patients with a new experimental treatment, while such patients were not excluded from the historical controls.

As an alternative one may introduce the new treatment at one hospital and continue using the old one at another hospital. That method, however, is also unreliable as one can never be certain that the patients are fully comparable and that the adjuvant therapy is identical.

Fibiger had realized these problems in 1898 [123] when he published the results of a controlled trial of the effect of an antitoxin in diphtheria during childhood. Four hundred and eighty-four children entered the trial which lasted for one year, serum treatment and no treatment being given on alternate days. He observed eight deaths in the treatment group compared with 30 deaths in the equally large control group. The methods may not have been perfect according to present-day standards, but the trial was unique in an international context, and Fibiger was far ahead of his time.

The breakthrough only occurred after the Second World War when the Medical Research Council promoted the use of controlled clinical trials. They refined the design by recommending random allocation of the patients to the different treatment groups, and this innovation greatly enhanced the reliability of the results. The streptomycin trial of pulmonary tuberculosis which was initiated by, among others, Bradford Hill was started in 1946 and the positive results were published two years later [124]. The negative results of new treatments which had initially been accepted uncritically, such as anticoagulant treatment of myocardial infarction and anticholinergic treatment of peptic ulcers, as well as the thalidomide affair in the 1960s, also paved the way to general acceptance of randomized clinical trials. The methods used today will be explained in the next chapter.

Alternative medicine: scientific and pseudoscientific thinking

This historical account might leave the impression that 'pseudoscientific' reasoning is now a thing of the past, and that at long last we have accepted that uncontrolled experience cannot be trusted and that all new treatments must be subjected to well-planned controlled trials. That, however, is not the case. Alternative medicine is flourishing, and it is as if many patients and even some doctors are actually attracted by its irrationality.

Here we shall not discuss all the bizarre offers of the alternative market, but there is much to choose between. Diagnoses are made by inspecting the patient's iris, by examining the patient's aura or by recording the propagation of the vibrations from a tuning fork placed on the knee. A large variety of herbs and special minerals are given as treatments, and so is application of magnetic or psychic force, the latter sometimes even at a distance. We encounter theories which superficially mimic scientific ones, and others which are associated with Eastern mysticism. We shall only mention a few of the more well-established schools.

We shall use the collective term alternative medicine although others prefer to talk about non-conventional or complementary medicine [125]. It is of course true that the various therapies are sometimes used as a complement to conventional medical treatment, but their theoretical foundation is so different from that of scientific medicine that it is truly alternative.

Homoeopathy was founded by Samuel Hahnemann towards the end of the eighteenth century. He developed the doctrine 'that like is cured by like' (*similia similibus curantur*), which is rooted in medieval medicine, and according to which patients presenting certain symptoms must be treated with those drugs which in healthy persons elicit similar symptoms. Thus, Hahnemann argued that in healthy persons quinine may provoke the symptoms of malaria and that therefore it acts curatively in that disease. A second doctrine is even more peculiar. It is held that infinitesimally small doses must be used, meaning that the preparation may be diluted so much that it is not certain that the patient ingests one single molecule. Homoeopaths are fully aware of this fact. They accept that the dilution may be beyond 'the Avogadro limit', but believe that the preparation has left some sort of imprint in the solvent [126,127]. Homoeopathy has never been very popular in Scandinavia, but thousands of homoeopaths practice in, for example, Great Britain, the United States and Germany.

Chiropractic is also a well-established school. It was founded in 1895 by Palmer, an American magnetic healer, and he believed that all diseases, including peptic ulcers, hypertension, diabetes, epilepsy, cancer and infections, were caused by small vertebral misalignments called subluxations [128]. Consequently, chiropractic therapy involves the detection and correction of these misalignments by means of manual manipulations, so-called 'adjustments'. Palmer's son treated infections with manipulations, and a little time spent surfing the Internet shows that chiropractic treatment is still used in children's asthma, hay fever, otitis and nocturnal enuresis. Some chiropractors claim that they confine themselves to the treatment of musculoskeletal diseases and that they accept the tradition of the natural sciences, but if they give up the idea of the pathogenic role of subluxations it is difficult to see the difference between chiropractic and physical medicine. A randomized trial of chiropractic treatment of patients with back pain showed only a marginal effect [129].

We shall also briefly mention *reflexology*, especially reflex zone therapy of the feet, which originated in the East and which has become very popular in some countries. It is believed that localized reflex points on the sole of the foot are connected with different parts of the body, and charts have been drawn showing the position of these points. Pressure applied on the right point is said to have a healing effect on the corresponding organ, be it the kidneys, the gall bladder or perhaps the heart.

When alternative therapists are asked why they believe that their treatments are so effective, they will invariably refer to their own personal experience and in some cases they may add that their treatment has ancient roots and that it would have been abandoned centuries ago if it was ineffective. These arguments are obviously invalid. We have already discussed in some detail the fallacies of uncontrolled experience, and ineffective treatments which originated in Greek Antiquity were used in Europe as late as the nineteenth century.

Many proponents of alternative practices also claim that their theories are holistic, i.e. take into account both the bodily and the spiritual aspects of the nature of man, whereas orthodox medicine is reductionistic, i.e. reduces man to a biological organism and endeavours to explain disease in physicochemical terms. These are difficult philosophical concepts, but in this context the use of the words seems mainly rhetorical. It is, for instance, difficult to imagine anything more 'reductionistic' than the theory that all kinds of diseases are caused by subluxations in the vertebral column. Nor does the idea that a wide spectrum of very different ailments can be cured by the intake of one particular mineral or by rubbing the soles of the feet seem particularly 'holistic'. It is, of course, to some extent true that medical science is reductionistic, but the clinician who seeks the physiological cause of the patient's symptoms need not ignore the ethical and hermeneutic aspects of the decision process (p. 147). Holism is a vague concept, and as yet no alternative school has suggested a credible theory which explains the age-old body–mind problem.

However, any discussion of the fundamental difference between alternative medicine and what we may call orthodox or scientific medicine presupposes that these terms have been defined, and that is not easy. Members of the medical profession debating this question often leave the impression that scientific medicine, almost by definition, is that which is practised by authorized medical doctors whereas alternative medicine is that which is practised by others. But this distinction is not tenable, as it is difficult to claim that medical doctors always reason scientifically and as some members of the medical profession even use 'alternative methods' in their clinical practice. Homoeopathic therapy does not become scientific because the drug is prescribed by an ill-advised medical doctor.

It is also unreasonable to claim that the theories of alternative medicine are always wrong, and that those of scientific medicine are always true. Admittedly, the alternative theories known to us are so much at variance with established knowledge that they must be regarded as false, but the theories of scientific medicine are not invulnerable. Undoubtedly, many of the theories found in the standard textbooks today will some time in the future be modified or rejected.

One might also suggest that alternative therapeutic practices are ineffective whereas those treatments that are used by medical doctors are effective.

This distinction is obviously unacceptable as there can be little doubt that medical practitioners use many ineffective treatments, and as some alternative treatments have considerable effects. Some herbal drugs sold as 'natural medicines' contain active substances with, for instance, antipyretic, anticholinergic or laxative effects and these effects are, of course, noticed by the patients. It is, however, difficult to see that it should be more 'natural' to take such drugs with an unknown content of a variety of substances, rather than taking an exact amount of a well-defined drug. Probably, most herbal drugs are quite harmless, but impurities may cause side-effects. Fatal illness has been reported after the intake of Chinese herbal tea [130].

The main difference between scientific and alternative medicine is rather more subtle; it reflects the difference between scientific and pseudoscientific thinking. Scientific thinking is characterized by a critical attitude to established theories on the part of the scientists. They seek weak points in the theories, generate new hypotheses and subject these to critical experiments. According to Popper, we must accept that our scientific theories are only approximations to the truth, and their 'verisimilitude' or trustworthiness depends on the zeal with which they have been exposed to critical experiments [131].

The proponents of alternative medicine do not reason like that. Reflexologists, for instance, do not test whether they have charted the position of the reflex points on the sole of the foot correctly, e.g. whether it makes any difference to patients with gall bladder disease if the pressure is applied to the 'kidney point' or *vice versa*, and homoeopaths do not expose their theory of '*similia similibus curantur*' to critical experiments. One proponent of homoeopathy even argued that it was one of the strengths of homoeopathy that it had not been changed. It was the same today as in Hahneman's days, whereas medical theories change all the time. The homoeopaths had found the truth [127].

It has been suggested that the efficacy of alternative treatments must be tested by means of randomized clinical trials, and that is in some cases a reasonable proposal. The theoretical rationale of an alternative practice may be fundamentally unsound, but it has often happened in the history of science that deductions from a false theory proved to be true. It is, for example, still a controversial issue whether or not acupuncture has an effect on pain, and more trials are needed, but, of course, the demonstration of an effect would not prove that the ancient Chinese theory of the 12 meridians is true. It would be necessary to explain the fact within the framework of our knowledge of physiological mechanisms. The hypothesis that acupuncture elicits the release of endomorphin has not been confirmed, but other suggestions have been made.

In other cases it may be taken for granted that both the theory and the deductions from the theory are false. Homoeopathic theory, for instance, is obviously untenable, and the deduction that drugs diluted beyond the Avogadro limit have any beneficial effects is equally unbelievable. Carrying out randomized trials must in this case be regarded as a somewhat futile exercise, as the acceptance of a result in favour of the treatment always requires a modicum of prior belief. Randomized trials where homoeopathic treatment is compared with no treatment have been done, and a meta-analysis revealed a general trend in favour of 'active' treatment [132]. This is an interesting study, but only because it reveals the importance of bias even in apparently well-controlled studies. We shall write more about this meta-analysis in the next chapter (p. 141).

In short, alternative medicine brings to mind the state of orthodox medicine in the eighteenth century when the age-old theory of the four humours and a variety of new, equally speculative theories of disease were flourishing. In those days medical practitioners, just like the proponents of alternative medicine today, believed that their uncontrolled experience confirmed the figments of their imagination. Alternative treatments are an anachronism in modern therapeutics.

CHAPTER 6

The Randomized Clinical Trial

Comparative experience is a prerequisite for experimental and
scientific medicine, otherwise the physician may walk at
random and become the sport of a thousand illusions.
[Claude Bernard [133]].

The half-life of medical knowledge is short and it is difficult for medical practitioners to keep up-to-date. The medical journals regularly publish the results of clinical studies which suggest that some new treatment is better than the current ones, and then it is not enough to read the abstract with the author's conclusions. The perfect scientific investigation has yet to be seen, and the critical reader must be well acquainted with the methodological pitfalls of clinical research.

The randomized clinical trial is the gold standard for the assessment of any treatment, not only pharmacotherapy, but also surgical interventions, physiotherapy, dietary treatment, different types of nursing care, and preventive measures in the general population. In this chapter we shall explain what we believe clinicians ought to know when they study the report of such a trial. Those who wish to do such trials themselves must seek additional information elsewhere [7].

Very often the standard design is used. A number of patients with the disease in question are allocated at random to two groups, the treatment group and the control group. The patients in the treatment group receive the new treatment, whereas those in the control group typically receive the treatment in current use. If possible, the trial is double-blind, which implies that neither patients nor investigator know to which group the individual patient belongs. The results of the two treatments are recorded and subjected to a statistical analysis. We shall now consider this design step by step.

Selection of patients

The 'Methods' section of the report of a randomized trial is sometimes written in small print, but it deserves special attention. The reader wishes to assess if he can use the results for the benefit of his own patients and, ideally, that requires the fulfilment of three conditions: the entry criteria must be well defined; the included patients must be a representative sample of all patients fulfilling the entry criteria; and the reader's own patients must be sufficiently similar to those in the trial.

It is a minimum requirement that the criteria for entry (symptoms, signs and paraclinical findings) and the criteria for exclusion (e.g. pregnancy, age limits or concomitant disease) are so well defined that the reader can recognize the patients. This means that he must be able to judge from the information in the paper which of his own patients would have entered the trial and which would not, because otherwise he cannot be sure to which patients he may apply the results of the study. Occasionally, the report only provides the information that a certain number of patients with, say, an irritable bowel syndrome or a myocardial infarction were included, and such trials are of limited value, as different clinicians use different diagnostic criteria for the diagnosis of these diseases.

Ideally, all patients fulfilling the entry criteria during the period of the trial should be enrolled, but that can rarely be achieved. It is, for instance, necessary to obtain the patients' informed consent, and some patients will probably refuse to take part. If, however, many patients fail to be included, the remainder may no longer constitute a representative sample of all patients fulfilling the entry criteria. The possible effect of such selection bias for the outcome of the trial depends on the clinical problem, and sometimes it cannot be ignored. If, for example, only 30% of those women with breast cancer who fulfilled the entry criteria had accepted participation in one of those trials which compared radical mastectomy and tumorectomy, it would have been very difficult to interpret the results. Perhaps women with palpable tumours refused to participate as they feared that the new treatment, tumorectomy, might not be as good as the old one, or perhaps those with a small nonpalpable tumour demonstrated by mammography did not want to lose their breast. Both types of bias are possible.

There is no perfect solution to this problem, apart from doing a subgroup analysis after the completion of the trial, comparing the treatment results in patients with palpable and nonpalpable tumours. If the results were the same, the importance of this particular factor would have been disproved. For these reasons reports of randomized trials ought to contain detailed information about eligible patients who were not enrolled, permitting the reader to judge for himself whether or not selection bias may have occurred. Much too often this information is missing.

The reader must also carefully consider to what extent his own patients resemble those of the trial. A general practitioner, for example, cannot take it for granted that he will obtain the same results as specialists at teaching hospitals, as his patients belong to a different part of the clinical spectrum. A new antidepressant which has been tested at a psychiatric hospital unit may not be equally effective in other settings. Geographical differences must also be taken into account. The frequency and manifestations of gastric cancer, for instance, are different in Japan compared with most European countries, and it cannot be excluded that the disease in these two parts of the world will respond differently to some new chemotherapy.

Randomization

The comparison of two treatments requires that everything possible has been done to ensure the comparability of the two groups of patients. As mentioned in the preceding chapter it is not sufficient to compare the results of a new treatment with those obtained previously or with those obtained at a different hospital, and unfortunately it is also impossible to let the patients themselves choose the treatment that they prefer. That suggestion was once made in connection with the breast cancer trials, but, for the reasons mentioned above, women with palpable cancers might have preferred mastectomy while those with nonpalpable ones might have chosen a tumorectomy. It would have been impossible to interpret the results.

The only solution to these difficulties is randomization. Random allocation to the two treatment groups effectively prevents systematic differences, but of course imbalances may still occur due to random variation. If the number of patients is small, it cannot be excluded that patients who for some reason or other have a poor prognosis, simply by chance, predominate in one of the treatment groups, but, if the sample is sufficiently large, different types of patients will tend to be evenly distributed in the two groups. However, imbalances arising at random are subject to the laws of chance, and a proper statistical analysis will tell to what extent they may have influenced the results of the trial. The necessary sample size is calculated before the start of the trial, and the method used must be stated in the resulting paper (see p. 189).

The randomization procedure is best explained by describing the method that was used prior to the introduction of computer technology and which is still sometimes used. At the planning stage a helper, who afterwards is not connected with the trial, produces the randomization sequence. If the sample size calculation has shown that 120 patients are needed, the helper may, in principle, toss a coin 120 times (having decided in advance that 'heads' = treatment *A* and 'tails' = treatment *B*) and write down the sequence, e.g. AABABBBAABABABAAB.... In practice, however, he will simulate the tosses, using random number tables or series of random numbers generated by a pocket calculator. Then the clinician running the trial, who of course does not see the list, receives a stack of 120 firmly closed, numbered envelopes, each containing a card marked treatment *A* or treatment *B*.

If it is a double-blind trial, which compares two drugs in tablet form, the clinician will also receive 120 numbered bottles, containing the right sort of tablets for each patient, and the envelopes will remain closed. If, on the other hand, the trial is open, e.g. a trial comparing a medical and a surgical treatment, the clinician must of course open the numbered envelopes in succession each time a new patient enters the trial, in order to see which treatment to give.

This procedure is fully acceptable, apart from the fact that it is not foolproof if somebody wants to cheat. It may be possible to read what is written on the card, if the envelope is held up to a bright light, and, if the trial is open and several patients are admitted on the same day, it is possible to open several envelopes at once and then decide which patient should have which treatment.

Therefore, randomization by computer is becoming the standard procedure. The clinical investigator enters the entry criteria, and if (and only if) these are fulfilled the computer program will allocate the patient at random to one of the treatment groups and provide a code number which tells the investigator which bottle to take. Then any suspicion of fraud is avoided.

Sometimes more elaborate randomization procedures are used in order to ensure that subgroups of patients are equally distributed in the two treatment groups. In large multicentre trials where each centre is expected to recruit, say, 10 patients, it may be useful to use *block randomization*, e.g. to randomize in blocks of 10, so that each centre provides five patients for the treatment group and five patients for the control group. One may also use randomization procedures which ensure that the two patient groups are comparable as regards severity of disease, length of history or some other factor of known or assumed prognostic significance. However, such prior subdivision or *stratification* of the patients makes a trial less easy to handle.

In the past more simple procedures were used. Sometimes the patients were allocated to the two treatments according to their date of birth (e.g. even date = new treatment and odd date = old treatment) or date of admission, but experience shows that the results of such trials must be interpreted with caution. In one trial which compared a surgical and a medical treatment, it was found afterwards that the average age of the surgically treated patients was lower than that of the medically treated ones. All patients who are considered bad risks from a surgical point of view, including those who are old and frail, must of course be excluded from a trial of this kind and, possibly, this exclusion criterion was treated more leniently among those who, according to their date of birth, were to receive medical treatment than among those who were to be treated surgically. Such bias can only be avoided if the following rule is applied: first it is decided whether the patient is eligible for the trial by fulfilling all the entry criteria, next it is determined by some random procedure which treatment the patient should be given.

It has been shown that trials in which the randomization procedure is not optimal tend to overestimate the effect of new treatments [134], and it is unfortunate that authors rarely report in detail which method they used.

Choice of treatment in the control group

According to the standard design, the patients in the treatment group receive the new treatment while those in the control group receive the one in current use. Obviously, this is the right procedure from the point of view of the clinician who wishes to know whether or not the new treatment is any better than the one already in use. He would not wish to change to the new treatment unless it is more effective, except perhaps in those cases where it is cheaper or has fewer side-effects.

Alternatively, one may compare the new treatment with no treatment, which means that the patients in the control group of a double-blind drug trial receive inert, dummy tablets. This design, however, is only acceptable from a clinical and an ethical point of view if no other effective treatment is available, in which case one may say that no treatment is the best current treatment. This is an important point as much of the criticism which has been raised against this type of research stems from the misconception that half the participating patients always receive inert tablets ('placebo tablets').

Representatives of the drug industry may, of course, take a different view of the matter. If they wish to register a new drug, they have to prove that it is effective, but not necessarily that it is more effective than those already on the market. Therefore, from their point of view it is sufficient to compare with inert tablets. They may also pay attention to the fact that a comparison of two effective drugs requires many more patients than a comparison with inert tablets. Such commercial interests are legitimate, but they are irrelevant from a clinical point of view.

Principles of blinding

Open trials where the doctor as well as the patient knows which treatment is given, always involve a considerable risk of bias. The doctor may be biased, having made up his mind in advance that the new treatment is best, and this belief may well influence the way in which he questions the patient and interprets the treatment result. The patients may also be biased as those who know that they are trying something new may have greater confidence in the effect than those who get the standard treatment, and this difference in expectations may induce different placebo effects.

It is well known that it is possible to eliminate psychological bias of that kind by doing a *double-blind trial*, but it is less appreciated that blinding also has other important advantages. If, for example, some patients develop unexpected symptoms or signs, such as dizziness, diarrhoea or a slight increase in liver enzymes, it is necessary to decide whether or not they should be withdrawn from the trial, and this decision may be biased if the trial is open. The clinician may decide to withdraw a patient on the suspicion of an unknown side-effect if he receives the new treatment, but ignore the observation if he belongs to the control group. As a result there would be more withdrawals due to suspected side-effects in the treatment group than in the control group. This problem does not arise in double-blind trials where the clinician is ignorant of the treatment given when the decision is made. If it is considered necessary, he may of course afterwards open the code for that particular patient and ascertain which treatment was given.

Sometimes it is necessary to use a more sophisticated design. Perhaps the two types of tablets differ in appearance or perhaps the dosage or time intervals differ. In that case it is necessary to manufacture dummy tablets looking like drug *A* and dummy tablets looking like drug *B*. Then it is possible to preserve blindness by using the so-called *double-dummy technique*, according to which the patients in one group receive drug *A* + dummy *B*, and those in the other drug *B* + dummy *A*.

The reader of the report should always ask himself whether or not the blinding was successful. Sometimes it is stated that the trial was double-blind when, in fact, in some cases either the patient or the doctor had guessed which treatment was given. One of the drugs may have an acid taste, discolour the urine or be associated with other characteristic effects. In one allegedly double-blind trial of peppermint oil capsules against irritable bowel symptoms, some of the patients reported that members of their family had noticed the smell of peppermint when they had used the w.c. Problems of this kind are particularly likely to occur in cross-over trials (see below) where the patients experience both treatments, and it is always advisable to ask all patients on their last visit what their guess is as regards the treatment they received.

The double-blind technique also requires modification if it is necessary to individualize the number of tablets given to each patient according to the treatment response. Oral anticoagulant treatment, for instance, requires frequent adjustment of the dose, for which reason the standard design cannot be used. Instead the trial is designed in such a way that one doctor, who has no personal contact with the patients, adjusts the dose of anticoagulant tablets in the actively treated patients and, in a similar fashion, alters the dosage of the dummy tablets in the control group. Then a different clinician may record the treatment effect without knowing to which treatment group the patients belong. Such trials may appropriately be called *double-blind with open therapeutic monitoring*.

A similar situation occurs when surgeons wish to compare two different surgical procedures. Here the surgeons cannot, of course, be 'blind', but the problem is solved if somebody else, for instance a physician, assesses the treatment result.

It would be much simpler to solve these problems by doing a *single-blind trial* where only the patients are kept 'blind', but, usually, the reliability of this design is little better than that of the open trial. The doctor may be biased when he assesses the treatment result and he may not induce the same placebo effect in the two treatment groups. In one trial, however, this problem was solved by letting the 'blind' patients, themselves, assess their condition. The trial compared laparoscopic cholecystectomy with small-incision cholecystectomy by laparotomy, and the patients and nurses were kept 'blind' as similar bandages were used in all cases. It is commonly believed that laparoscopic surgery, although it takes longer, has the advantage that the patients can be discharged from hospital much earlier, but in this trial where the 'blind' patients decided for themselves when they felt ready to go home, the length of the hospital stay was the same in the two groups [135].

In general, single-blind trials where the doctor, but not the patient, is 'blind' are more useful. When, for instance, the effect of two training programmes for back pain are compared, it is not possible to conceal the nature of the treatment from the patient, but the doctor who assesses the treatment result need not know which treatment was given.

It follows from this discussion that often it is not possible to do the perfect double-blind trial, and in all such cases the investigators can do no more than choose that technique which reduces the risk of bias as much as is at all possible. If it is necessary to do an open trial it may still be feasible to blind part of the assessment, e.g. the reading of X-ray films or the physical examination of the patient. The risk of bias depends on the measures of effect and thus it varies from trial to trial. The patients' own assessment of their subjective symptoms is of course much more sensitive to bias than determinations of survival time or other objective observations but, unfortunately, the objective measures of effect may sometimes be less relevant from a clinical point of view than the subjective ones.

Both randomization and blinding are very important tools for the prevention of bias, and of these the former is the more important. Randomization can always be done properly whereas perfect blinding is an ideal which sometimes can be attained, especially in drug trials.

Cross-over trials

The design which has been discussed so far is the group comparative trial, where the patients are allocated to a treatment group and a control group. If, however, the disease is of long duration, and if the treatment only alleviates the symptoms, but does not alter the course of the disease, it may be worthwhile to design a cross-over trial where each patient provides his own control. According to that design all patients are given both treatments, the old drug and the new drug, in succession, and the response to the two treatments is recorded and compared. This kind of trial also requires randomization, ensuring that the treatment order varies at random, and, if possible, blinding so that neither doctor nor patient knows which treatment is given during which period.

The interval between the administration of the drug and the onset of effect must be short and the effect must subside quickly after cessation of medication, i.e. there must be no *carry-over effect* to the next treatment period. In cross-over trials comparing an active drug (A) and a dummy preparation (B), the carry-over phenomenon will have the effect that the 'response' to treatment B is larger in those patients who receive treatment B after treatment A than in those who receive treatment B before treatment A. A wash-out period between the two treatment periods may solve the problem, but the trial becomes more laborious and the risk of drop-outs increases.

It is usually stated that cross-over trials require fewer patients than group comparative trials, since the patients serve as their own controls and the between-patient variation has been eliminated. Sometimes, however, the situation is not that simple. In some conditions the symptoms fluctuate so much that the between-period variation in individual patients is almost as large as the between-patient variation in groups of patients, and if that is the case the simpler group comparative design is to be preferred.

It must also be remembered that patients with chronic diseases usually turn to their doctor when their symptoms are at their worst, and therefore it is often seen that the patients' symptoms tend to improve during the second treatment period, regardless of the treatment given. This phenomenon is called a *period effect*. Occasionally the reports of cross-over trials are so detailed that it is possible for the reader to detect carry-over or period effects which were overlooked by the authors.

The choice of outcome measures

The clinical data which serve to measure the treatment effects must be as reliable as possible, as regards both their reproducibility and their accuracy, and, first of all, they must be clinically relevant. This topic, which was discussed in some detail in Chapter 2, is of particular importance for the planning and interpretation of randomized clinical trials.

In many trials the choice of outcome measures is uncontroversial. Antiviral drugs used for the treatment of herpes zoster must be tested for their effects on the pain and the rash, and in trials with antiepileptic drugs one must consider the frequency and severity of epileptic fits. In other studies, however, the situation is rather more complex. In trials of cancer chemotherapy, for instance, it is not sufficient to determine the survival time. One must also record the occurrence and severity of a variety of symptoms, both those caused by the disease and those caused by the treatment, and global assessments of the patients' clinical condition may be appropriate, preferably using simple rating scales.

Clinical research workers sometimes show considerable ingenuity when they choose the outcome measures, and they may go too far. In trials of antirheumatic drugs, patients are often asked to squeeze the inflated cuff of a sphygmomanometer to permit the measurement of grip strength in mmHg. Perhaps it is found that one drug causes a greater increase in the grip strength than the other and perhaps this difference is statistically significant (see below), but it is by no means certain that an increase from, say, 120–140 mmHg has any clinical significance whatsoever. It might have been better to focus on the patients' ability to cope with their daily chores. Other irrelevant effect measures in arthritis trials were mentioned on page 19.

Sometimes *surrogate outcome measures* are used, i.e. outcome measures which are not clinically relevant *per se*, but are believed to be good indicators of the clinically relevant outcome, and this may be justified in some cases. At present, for example, gastroenterologists test different drug combinations for the eradication of *Helicobacter pylori* in patients with duodenal ulcer. Usually, the *Helicobacter* infection causes no symptoms at all, and the true aim of the treatment is to prevent ulcer recurrence. Therefore, successful eradication is a surrogate outcome, but it is an acceptable one as it has been shown in other studies that ulcer recurrences in *Helicobacter*-negative persons are extremely rare.

In other cases the use of surrogate outcomes is more doubtful [136]. We have already mentioned (p. 37) the trial of fluoride treatment in cases of osteoporosis where the bone mineral content served as a surrogate outcome in the belief that an increased content would lower the risk of fractures. However, fluoride treatment which had the desired effect on the surrogate outcome also led to an increased risk of fractures.

The lowering of the blood pressure in short-term trials of antihypertensive drugs against mild hypertension may also be regarded as a surrogate outcome, as the patients have no symptoms at all. The true aim of the treatment is to lower the future risk of cerebrovascular and cardiovascular incidents, and the normalization of the blood pressure may well serve this purpose, but the possible adverse effect of long-term treatment must not be ignored. It has, for instance, been suggested that treatment with short-acting calcium channel-blocking agents is accompanied by an increase in the risk of myocardial infarction [137].

The introduction of new antiarrhythmic drugs in the 1980s is the most frightening example of the dire results of using a surrogate measure. Certain types of ventricular dysrhythmias arising after a myocardial infarction predispose to ventricular fibrillation and death from cardiogenic shock. Therefore, it was taken for granted that the new drugs, which in randomized trials were found to restore the normal cardiac rhythm in patients with dysrhythmia, would also prevent sudden cardiac deaths, and soon they were widely used after an acute myocardial infarction. However, a number of unexpected deaths raised the suspicion that the drugs were not safe, and finally they were tested in a randomized clinical trial where the end-point was not the immediate antiarrhythmic effect, but the effect on survival. It turned out that in some patients the drugs produced arrhythmias and the net result of their use was that the risk of death rose rather than fell [138,139]. The treatment was used extensively in the United States and it has been estimated that it caused the death of more than 50 000 people per year in that country alone, i.e. more than the American loss of lives during the Vietnam War.

These examples illustrate that the interaction between disease mechanisms and the mechanisms of action of different drugs is so complex that it is dangerous not to record directly the clinically relevant outcomes. However, it is easy to understand that clinical research workers often feel tempted to use surrogate measures. The effect of an antihypertensive drug on the blood pressure is seen after a few weeks, and relatively few patients with dysrhythmia are needed to ascertain that a drug has an antiarrhythmic effect. Much longer follow-up periods and many more patients are required to record the clinically relevant effect on prognosis and survival.

Sometimes the distinction between surrogate measures and clinically relevant outcomes is not quite simple. It is, for instance, well established that bronchoconstriction plays a causal role in acute asthma, and therefore it may be reasonable to use the results of spirometry as measures of effect in trials of different bronchodilators. Even in this case, however, many clinicians drew the wrong conclusions. They overlooked that the trials only showed that the drugs were effective in an acute attack, and that the results did not support the use of long-term treatment. Previously, it was customary, at least in some countries, to advise asthma patients to use their inhaler four times daily regardless of their clinical condition. Now it is generally accepted that intermittent asthma only requires bronchodilatory treatment on an 'as needed' basis [140].

Papers reporting randomized trials must also provide information about adverse effects. Patients taking part in double-blind trials will be monitored regularly both by careful questioning and by paraclinical tests, e.g. blood and urine analyses aimed at detecting damage to the liver, kidney or bone marrow. Usually, some participants in randomized trials complain of mild symptoms, such as headache, dyspepsia, diarrhoea or dizziness, and the frequency of these complaints may well be the same in the treatment group and in a control group where the patients only receive inert tablets. Nevertheless careful monitoring is essential as the testing of new drugs is always associated with a risk of serious side-effects. All subjective symptoms must be recorded, and their severity must be noted.

The sample size of a randomized clinical trial must be so large that clinically significant, beneficial effects are not likely to be missed, but it is rarely large enough to guarantee the detection of rare adverse effects. Drug treatment of a trivial disease is of course quite unacceptable if one patient in four hundred experiences a serious side-effect, but a simple calculation will show that there is only a 30% probability that this event will occur if the treatment group comprises 500 patients. Therefore, it is very important that medical practitioners watch out for all unexpected events when they start using a new drug and that they report these to the relevant authority.

Stopping rules

It must be decided in advance when a randomized trial is to stop, i.e. when no more patients are to be admitted. The correct procedure is to declare the necessary sample size in the protocol and to stop the trial when that number of patients has been reached. Otherwise, if the trial is not 'blind', the investigators may be tempted to look at the results in the two treatment groups from time to time and then stop the trial when they feel convinced that the new treatment is better than the old one. That is of course quite impermissible. If two treatments are equally effective and if the results in the two groups are compared repeatedly throughout the trial, it is only to be expected that the new treatment from time to time, simply by chance, will have provided better results than the old one. To conclude the trial when that has happened is equivalent to the introduction of new rules for the next soccer game between England and Denmark: the game is stopped as soon as Denmark is in the lead, but it continues if the two teams are even, or if England is in the lead. Undoubtedly, the English supporters would object strongly to this idea. Unfortunately, those clinical research workers who use that kind of stopping rule are unlikely to write it in their paper, and the reader of the article will be misled.

But there is no rule without exceptions. It may be desirable for ethical reasons to ensure that the trial can be stopped prematurely, if the difference between the treatment results in the two groups proves to be particularly large or if one of the treatments causes serious adverse effects. That possibility must, however, be foreseen at the planning stage by the establishment of an independent safety committee, i.e. a committee of experts not associated with the running of the trial, who have access to the randomization code and may look at the results at regular intervals. However, the decision to stop the trial should not just be left to the discretion of that committee. Ideally, it must be stated in the protocol which statistical calculations they should do (usually a so-called group sequential analysis) and under which circumstances they are authorized to 'pull the emergency cord'.

Assessment of the results

The assessment of the results after the completion of the trial invariably involves subjective judgements. The inspection of the information about each individual patient will probably reveal that some of them did not fulfil the requirements of the protocol, as some may have missed one or more of the stipulated visits to the research clinician while others did not take the drug as prescribed. There can be no doubt that those patients who simply did not complete the trial or did not take the tablets at all must be recorded as drop-outs, but in other cases it is a matter of choice whether or not the patient should be labelled as such. Therefore, in order to prevent bias, those who make the decisions ought not know to which treatment group the patients belong, but unfortunately this rule has not yet gained general acceptance. A survey of randomized trials of antirheumatic drugs revealed many examples of bias in connection with the analysis and the interpretation of the results, usually in favour of the new drug [38].

The inspection of the database is followed by the numerical analysis of the results, which in some trials simply amounts to calculating the cure rate in the two treatment groups. The handling of the drop-outs may, however, cause serious problems. The simplest solution is to do a *per protocol analysis* which only includes those patients who completed the trial as planned, but the exclusion of the drop-outs may be a cause of bias. Perhaps some of those patients who received the new treatment did not turn up for the scheduled visits because the treatment did not help them at all or perhaps they felt so well that the visits did not seem worthwhile. It is possible both to overrate and to underrate the treatment effect.

The *intention-to-treat analysis* was introduced to solve this problem. Here all patients who entered the two treatment groups are included, whether or not they completed the trial according to the protocol. This type of analysis is realistic if it is possible to record the outcome in all patients, including the drop-outs. That was the case in a large trial of acetylsalicylic acid, given to patients with atrial fibrillation in order to prevent major cerebrovascular accidents, where all cases of stroke, including those among the drop-outs, could be retrieved by means of various registers. In the majority of trials, however, this is not possible. Some years ago numerous trials were done, which compared the effect of different H_2-blockers and proton pump inhibitors on the healing of peptic ulcers, and one could not possibly know whether or not the ulcer had healed if the patient did not turn up for the gastroscopy at the end of treatment. Usually, it was assumed in the intention-to-treat analyses that the ulcer had remained unhealed in all drop-outs, and obviously that assumption was unwarranted. In order to be on the safe side, the clinician might have made the assumption that the ulcers of the drop-outs in the treatment group had remained unhealed whereas those in the control group had healed. In practice, it may be necessary to do both a per protocol analysis and several intention-to-treat analyses, making different assumptions. If the results of these analyses differ too much, it may be necessary to conclude that the number of drop-outs was so large that the trial was a failure.

The statistical analysis

Hypothesis testing

It is not sufficient to quote the cure rate in each treatment group. The results must be subjected to a statistical analysis in order to assess the possible influence of random variation, and the principle is best explained by means of a numerical example.

Table 10a shows the results of a group comparative trial with 300 patients in each treatment group. Two hundred and forty, or 80%, of those patients who received drug *A* were cured compared with 210, or 70%, of those who were treated with drug *B*. Consequently, the difference between the cure rates is 10%. These results suggest that treatment *A* is more efficient than treatment

Table 10 Results of three randomized trials.

(a)

	Cured	Not cured	*Total*
Treatment *A*	240	60	*300*
Treatment *B*	210	90	*300*
Total	*450*	*150*	*600*

(b)

	Cured	Not cured	*Total*
Treatment *A*	233	67	*300*
Treatment *B*	210	90	*300*
Total	*443*	*157*	*600*

(c)

	Cured	Not cured	*Total*
Treatment *A*	226	74	*300*
Treatment *B*	210	90	*300*
Total	*436*	*164*	*600*

B, but we cannot exclude the possibility that they are in fact equally effective and that the difference arose by chance.

The statistical analysis of the results of the trial begins with the formulation of two hypotheses, which are denoted the *null hypothesis* and the *alternative hypothesis*. According to the null hypothesis, the two treatments are equally good (the observed difference between the results is due to random variation) and, according to the alternative hypothesis, treatment A is better than treatment B. The third logical possibility that treatment B is better than treatment A seems rather unlikely in this case and we shall choose to ignore it. The clinician who has to make the choice between treatment A and treatment B cannot know which of the two hypotheses is true, but in spite of that he has to make up his mind which treatment he is going to prescribe in the future. The situation is illustrated by Table 11, in which H_0 denotes the null hypothesis and H_A the alternative hypothesis. It is seen that there are four possibilities depending on the truth and the clinician's choice.

1   The physician decides to act as if the two treatments are equally good, and the two treatments are equally good. He accepts a true null hypothesis and commits no error.

2   The physician decides to act as if treatment A is better than treatment B, but the truth is that the two treatments are equally good. He rejects a true null hypothesis, and consequently he makes a mistake. In statistical terminology this mistake is called a *type I error* (an error of the first kind, or an α-error).

3   The physician decides to act as if the two treatments are equally good, but the truth is that treatment A is better than treatment B. He accepts a false null hypothesis, and in statistical terms he is committing a *type II error* (an error of the second kind, or a β-error).

4   The physician decides to act as if treatment A is better than treatment B, and treatment A is better than treatment B. He rejects a false null hypothesis and commits no error.

Table 11 Type I and type II errors.

		Truth	
		H_A: A ≠ B	H_0: A = B
Physician's choice	H_A: A ≠ B	No error	Type I error
	H_0: A = B	Type II error	No error

The distinction between type I and type II errors is important, but admittedly it is rather difficult to remember which is which. Perhaps the following mnemonic will be of some help. A doctor studies the results of a randomized trial and wonders whether or not he should reject the null hypothesis that the new treatment is no better than the old one. If he is an optimist he will be easily convinced, and if the null hypothesis is true he will have committed a type I error. If, however, he is a pessimist he may be more difficult to convince and he may stick to the null hypothesis in spite of the fact that the new drug is better. Then he is committing a type II error. O precedes P as I precedes II, and therefore the 'optimist error' is a type I error and the 'pessimist error' is a type II error.

It now remains to consider to what extent the actual results of the trial are compatible with the two hypotheses, H_0 and H_A, and for this purpose it is customary to do a suitable *significance test*. Here we shall not discuss the mathematics of the tests, but the procedure is as follows: we make the assumption that the two treatments are identical, i.e. that the null hypothesis is true, and then we calculate the probability of obtaining, by chance, a difference between the treatment results which, numerically, is as large or larger than the one observed in the trial. The choice of the statistical test depends on the problem at hand (see Chapter 8), and in this case it would be appropriate to use Fisher's exact test (or a χ^2 -test). We shall find that $P = 0.006$, and this result must be interpreted as follows: The probability (P) of obtaining a difference between the cure rates of 10% or more, either in favour of treatment A or in favour of treatment B, if the null hypothesis were true, is less than 0.006, i.e. less than 1%. Perhaps the clinician would feel that this chance is so small that he must act as if the alternative hypothesis is the true one, but he cannot be absolutely certain that he is right and he may be committing a type I error.

The other two examples in Table 10 can be analysed in exactly the same manner. If treatment A had cured seven less patients (Table 10b) the difference between the two cure rates would only have been 8%, and the statistical analysis would have shown that $P = 0.04$, i.e. that the chance of obtaining at least such a difference, if the null hypothesis were true, would be 4%. In the third example (Table 10c), the number of patients cured by treatment A has once again been reduced by seven, and now the difference between the cure rates is only 5%. The P-value would be 0.17, i.e. there would be a 17% probability of obtaining at least such a difference, if the treatments were in fact equally effective. Under those circumstances the clinician might decide to act as if the null hypothesis were true, and by doing so he would either be right or he would be committing a type II error.

According to convention, a difference is said to be statistically significant, if the P-value is less than 5%. Therefore, we may say that treatment *A* gave significantly better results than treatment *B* in the first two examples, but not in the third, and it is often implied by these expressions that in the first two examples the clinician ought to accept that the new treatment is more effective, whereas in the third he ought to accept the null hypothesis. Sometimes it is almost regarded as 'unscientific' to believe in a result which is statistically non-significant, or not to believe in one which is statistically significant. This convention, however, is most unfortunate, as it may well lead to a mental block which prevents the correct interpretation of the calculated P-values. This important point is best explained by an example.

Imagine that we hear about a trial which compares the effect of tablets made from a particular herb and inert tablets on the survival time of patients suffering from a particular kind of cancer. We are well acquainted with the literature on the topic and the available scientific evidence makes us conclude that there is only one chance in a thousand that the herb is effective. In other words, we attribute the alternative hypothesis a probability of 0.1%. Then imagine that the trial is completed and that the results are those shown in Table 10b. The difference is statistically 'significant' as the P-value is slightly less than 5%, but irrespective of that result we should not suddenly change our minds and conclude that the herb is effective. Our prior confidence in the alternative hypothesis was only 0.1%, and we should not be convinced by a result which is likely to occur in almost 5% of trials when the null hypothesis is true.

This problem is analogous to the one which was discussed on page 103 in connection with the interpretation of confidence intervals and it shows that we must distinguish between frequential (statistical) probabilities and subjective probabilities. The statistician asks the following question, 'What is the frequential probability of obtaining the observed results (or even more extreme results), if the null hypothesis is true?', and the P-value is the answer.

The reader of the medical journal who has to make up his mind whether or not to believe in the efficacy of the drug asks the reverse question: what is the probability that the null hypothesis is true, now that I have seen the reported results? This is a subjective probability and it depends not only on the P-value, but also on one's prior confidence in the null hypothesis and the alternative hypothesis.

Attempts have been made to formalize this type of reasoning (by means of so-called Bayesian statistics), but here we shall only suggest a simple rule-of-thumb: one should not reject the null hypothesis, if the *P*-value is larger than our prior confidence in the alternative hypothesis.

However, the decision not to be persuaded by the result does not necessarily imply that it should be ignored. If, later, we read about other studies which have a similar outcome, we shall remember the results in the previous reports. Gradually our prior confidence in the alternative hypothesis will increase and in the end we shall feel convinced that it is true.

Similar reasoning is appropriate if the statistical analysis resulted in a non-significant *P*-value and if our prior confidence in the alternative hypothesis was high. This might be the case if the new drug had already been shown to possess the same biological properties as other similar drugs which are effective. If the number of patients is small, we may decide, in spite of a large *P*-value, that probably the treatment is effective and that we should commit a type II error if we concluded otherwise. In Chapter 8 (pp. 190–3) these arguments will be illustrated by a numerical example.

P-values are frequently misinterpreted, and some doctors even mistake statistical significance for clinical significance. They believe that a small *P*-value (high statistical significance) is equivalent to a large clinical effect, and that a high *P*-value indicates that a treatment is less effective. That is, of course, a misunderstanding. If Table 10a showed the effect of two treatments on the survival of patients with a malignant disease, we should say that the difference was highly significant from a clinical point of view, whereas we should be less impressed if it showed the difference between the antipruritic effect of two ointments for haemorrhoids. The importance of a given difference depends on the clinical problem. It should also be born in mind that a difference between the treatment effects in the two groups will become statistically significant, no matter how small it is, if only the number of patients is sufficiently large.

Estimation

Conventional significance tests have the limitation that they only help the clinician to decide whether or not the effect of a new treatment differs from that of an old one. They do not answer the question: How much better (or how much worse) is the new treatment? In order to extract that information from the results of a randomized trial, we shall have to estimate the therapeutic gain or, in other words, we must calculate the 95% confidence interval of the observed difference [141].

Consider once again the first of the three numerical examples (Table 10a) where the observed difference between the treatment effects, i.e. the observed therapeutic gain, was 10%. The calculation of the 95% confidence interval of an observed rate was mentioned on pp. 102–6, and the 95% confidence interval of the difference between two rates can be calculated in much the same way. In this case it will be found that the 95% confidence interval is 3% to 17% which suggests that the therapeutic gain is at least 3% and at most 17%. However, the calculated confidence interval only includes the true therapeutic gain in 19 out of 20 trials, and, when judging the results of a particular trial, we should always consider the possibility that we are faced with the 'twentieth trial' where the true therapeutic gain is lower than the lower confidence limit or higher than the higher limit. The results of other studies or other kinds of information may suggest that this is the case.

In the example in Table 10b the observed therapeutic gain had been reduced to 8%, and a calculation will show that now the 95% confidence interval is 1% to 15%. Therefore, according to this calculation, the therapeutic gain is at least 1% and at most 15%. In Table 10c the therapeutic gain is even smaller, i.e. 5%, and the 95% confidence interval is –2% to 12%. This means that by using treatment A instead of treatment B one may expect to cure between 2% fewer patients and 12% more patients.

The confidence intervals agree well with the P-values, which was only to be expected as the calculations are based on similar principles. In the first two examples the interval did not include 0%, and the P-value was statistically significant ($P < 0.05$); both results suggest that the null hypothesis should be rejected. In the third example the interval included 0% and the P-value was statistically nonsignificant, suggesting that the null hypothesis should not be rejected.

The calculated confidence intervals of the therapeutic gain are especially revealing if the number of patients is small. Imagine a randomized trial of 60 patients where 15 of 30 patients who received treatment A were cured compared with 12 of 30 patients who received treatment B. The therapeutic gain is 10%, just as in Table 10a, but now it will be found that the 95% confidence interval is –15% to 35%. According to this calculation treatment A may cure up to 35% more patients than treatment B, but it is not excluded that it cures 15% fewer patients. A significance test would only show that the null hypothesis might well be true, i.e. that the two treatments might be identical, but it provides no information as regards the possible size of the difference.

Today most leading medical journals, e.g. the *British Medical Journal* [142,143], require that the authors quote the confidence intervals, and not only the P-values, but sometimes the reader may wish to calculate the intervals himself. That is easily done (with some approximation) using the following formula:

$$TG \pm 2 \sqrt{\frac{p_1(1-p_1)}{N_1} + \frac{p_2(1-p_2)}{N_2}}$$

where p_1 and p_2 are the cure rates and N_1 and N_2 the number of patients in each group. TG is the therapeutic gain $(p_1 - p_2)$.

Other statistical measures of effect

The therapeutic gain, i.e. the difference between the two cure rates, is the most relevant statistical measure of effect from a clinical point of view, but there are also other possibilities.

When, as in this case, we are dealing with data on a binomial scale (cured/not cured) one may also calculate the *relative risk* (RR). This statistical measure, which in recent years has become very popular, was first used in randomized clinical trials of treatments which served to prevent death (e.g. after a myocardial infarction) where it seemed more natural to talk about the 'risk of death' than the 'cure rate'. Now the RR is also calculated in other types of randomized trials. If, once again, we look at the figures in Table 10a it will be noted that the risk of *not* being cured was 20% in treatment group A and 30% in group B, and consequently the relative risk in favour of treatment A was 0.20/0.30 = 0.67. One may also calculate the confidence interval or do a significance test in order to assess whether the observed relative risk differs significantly from 1.

In spite of its popularity this statistical measure is unsatisfactory from a clinical point of view. A relative risk of 0.67 does not tell us whether the risk of not being cured (as in this case) was reduced from 30% to 20% or whether it was reduced from, say, 3% to 2%. In order to remedy this deficiency, it has been suggested that one should also calculate the *number needed to treat* (or *NNT*) [144], i.e. the number of patients who must be treated in order to cure (or save the life) of one patient. This number is simply the reciprocal of the therapeutic gain (or risk difference). Thus, NNT = 1/0.1 = 10, if the risk is reduced from 30% to 20%, and NNT = 1/0.01 = 100, if the risk is reduced from 3% to 2%. The number needed to treat may also be calculated directly from the figures in the fourfold table. Table 10a shows that 30 more patients were cured in group A than in group B. The number of patients in each group was 300, which means that it was necessary to treat 10 patients with treatment A in order to obtain one additional cure.

Effects measured on an ordinal or an interval scale require other statistical methods (see Chapter 8). Life table statistics are used to assess the survival time using different treatments (p. 20).

Subgroup analyses

When a randomized clinical trial has been completed, it is tempting to 'go fishing'. The total sample of patients is divided up into subgroups and the effect of the two treatments is compared for women alone, for men, for patients with particular symptoms, for old people, etc. That, of course, is a doubtful undertaking as, predictably, one in 20 of such subgroup comparisons will turn out to be statistically significant simply by chance, even when the null hypothesis is true. Further, subgroup analyses do not only invite type I errors, but also type II errors. If the trial as a whole revealed a difference between the treatment results, it cannot be expected that this difference will repeat itself in all subgroups.

Nevertheless, papers in medical journals frequently report the results of such 'fishing expeditions' which may well influence the clinical recommendations which are derived from the study. One large trial of the effect of streptokinase in acute myocardial infarction revealed a reduction of the death rate by 20%, but unfortunately the authors did a subgroup analysis and concluded that the treatment was only effective if it was started within 6 h of the onset of symptoms, and if the patient was younger than 65 years old and had an anterior infarction [145]. As usual, the conclusions derived from the fishing expedition were later disproved. The authors of a similar mega-trial were so annoyed by such conclusions that they added the result of an astrological subgroup analysis. They noted a decrease in the death rate in the trial as a whole, but added that the treatment was harmful to patients born under the sign of Gemini or Libra [146].

Meta-analysis

The impact of randomized clinical trials on patient management depends on the dissemination of the results within the medical profession. This is a process of great complexity which in recent years has attracted considerable attention.

The individual physician seeks to keep his knowledge up-to-date by reading his medical journals, and nowadays these contain an increasing number of reports of randomized trials. It is exciting to read that some new treatment is more effective than the one in current use, and, if the trial is sufficiently large and methodologically acceptable, it may be justified to adopt the new treatment immediately. Usually, however, a certain amount of healthy scepticism is in its place, as it cannot be excluded that some other journal, not read by the physician, reported another trial which gave a different result.

Therefore, it is also important to read good review articles written by experts who have done a thorough study of the literature in a particular field, but even that kind of information is not always trustworthy. It has been shown repeatedly that some reviews, even in the best medical journals, are biased, as the authors tend to quote only those papers which support their own point of view. Apart from that, even those authors who try to review the literature as objectively as possible must take into account the occurrence of *publication bias* [147], i.e. the phenomenon that trials with a statistically significant result are more likely to be published than those with a non-significant result. Usually, the results of large trials of a high methodological standard will reach the medical journals, regardless of the outcome, but smaller trials, especially those which gave a negative result, may not do so. If the outcome seems uninteresting, the investigators may not feel that it is worthwhile making the effort to analyse their data and to write a paper.

It has also been shown that trials done in non-English-speaking countries tend to be published in the national journals if the results are negative, and in international journals, written in English, if they are positive [148]. That was perhaps only to be expected, as those journals which enjoy the highest international reputation receive so many papers that they can permit themselves to be very selective. They naturally favour good papers with novel, unexpected scientific findings, and paradoxically that may well have the effect that the conclusions in those journals comprise more type I errors than those in the less prestigious ones.

All these circumstances suggest that there is a need for a research effort on a higher level, i.e. a research effort, the object of which is the research done by others. Such studies are called *meta-analyses* [149], if they include a comprehensive statistical analysis of the available evidence.

Each meta-analysis aims at creating a comprehensive and unbiased picture of the results of all those randomized clinical trials which address a particular clinical problem. It is a research project in its own right and, like other projects, it requires meticulous planning and a detailed protocol. The search of the literature is crucial as an attempt must be made to find all relevant studies, and the methods used must be described in detail in the final report. Then the reader may judge for himself whether or not it was sufficiently thorough. Commercial databases, such as MEDLINE, are essential sources of information, but their use requires considerable skill, and usually an iterative search strategy is needed, where some of the words from the titles and abstracts of the first papers to be retrieved are used for a renewed search. In spite of such efforts, the MEDLINE system may only ensure the retrieval of about 50% of those reports which have been published, and it is also necessary to use other sources of information, especially the Cochrane database which is mentioned below. In addition, unpublished studies may provide useful information, and it may be necessary to write to individual clinicians and to pharmaceutical companies known to be active in that particular area. Unfortunately the drug industry is not always very co-operative.

Figure 18 illustrates graphically the result of a meta-analysis based on 14 randomized clinical trials comparing two treatments, A and B, of a particular disease. The therapeutic gain (the difference between the cure rates in the two treatment groups) and the 95% confidence interval for the therapeutic gain are shown for each trial. The width of the confidence interval reflects the sample size, which in this analysis varied between 80 and 800; the larger the number of patients, the smaller the interval.

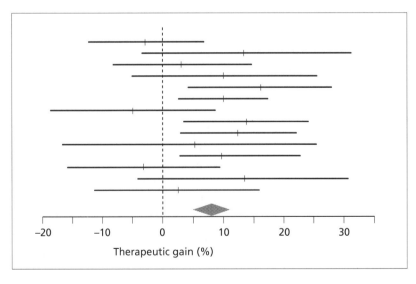

Fig. 18 The result of a meta-analysis of 14 randomized trials comparing two treatments, A and B. For each trial the therapeutic gain is shown (the difference between the cure rates in the two treatment groups) and the 95% confidence interval of this difference. The meta-analysis, combining the results of all 14 trials, revealed a therapeutic gain of 8% (95% confidence interval 5% to 11%) as illustrated by the diamond at the bottom of the graph.

It is seen that the best results were obtained with treatment *A* in 11 trials and with treatment *B* in three trials, but it is also seen that in nine trials the difference was statistically non-significant, as the confidence interval included 0%. It is possible to do a combined statistical analysis of all the trials, taking into account the differences in sample size, and in this case that kind of analysis revealed a therapeutic gain in favour of treatment *A* of 8% (95% confidence interval 5% to 11%). It is also possible to do a combined significance test, which in this meta-analysis gave the result $P < 0.00001$. In this case the meta-analyst calculated the combined therapeutic gain, but sometimes only the combined odds ratio (see p. 177) is reported. That measure of effect has statistical advantages, but it is very difficult to interpret from a clinical point of view.

If the number of trials is sufficiently large, it is also useful to look at the distribution of the results. It is only to be expected that the observed therapeutic gain will vary from trial to trial, and that the results of smaller trials will show greater variation than those of larger trials, but the distribution of the results will be symmetrical if the variation is purely random. If, however, the sample of trials included in the meta-analysis is biased, the distribution will be asymmetrical. Skewness to the right suggests publication bias caused by the fact that some negative trials never reached the medical journals [150].

Meta-analyses present many other difficulties which must be foreseen and addressed in the protocol. Methodologically flawed trials must be excluded, the criteria for the assessment of their quality having been specified in advance, and it must be decided whether the trials are sufficiently comparable to include them in the same statistical analysis. Otherwise the sample of trials must be subdivided into subgroups. Meta-analysts also face the problem that the reporting of randomized trials is not sufficiently standardized as regards, for instance, the choice of statistical methods [151]. However, the most important feature of a meta-analysis is not the statistical calculations, but the systematic search of the literature. Even without the combined statistical analysis the study can be published as a systematic review [152], which is much more valuable than the ordinary review articles.

The meta-analytic approach to therapeutic research was developed during the 1980s, and in 1993 the Cochrane Collaboration was established in order to promote the production of meta-analyses and systematic reviews. These are then published in the electronic Cochrane Database which is updated regularly [153]. The initiative was British, but in 1998 there were 15 Cochrane Centres in different parts of the world and 40 international multi-disciplinary groups that were busy hand-searching numerous medical journals in order to identify all published trials and to synthesize the available evidence. Anybody who is sufficiently qualified can join the collaboration, but those who accept to do systematic reviews are expected to update these when new trials appear.

The database now contains a large number of systematic reviews and proper meta-analyses, as well as more than 250 000 references to controlled trials. Therefore, the database is already so comprehensive that it should be consulted by any clinician who in his daily work wishes to assess the available knowledge about a particular treatment.

Meta-analysis, which combines the tradition of clinical research and modern information technology, is an efficient tool for assessing the aggregate knowledge of the effectiveness of a particular treatment at a given moment, but it is, of course, not infallible. There may be hidden sources of bias in the individual trial which cannot be detected even by careful reading of the report, and publication bias can never be fully excluded. Sometimes two meta-analyses of the same treatment have yielded different results, but usually it will be found that one of them was methodologically deficient in one way or another.

A recent example illustrates particularly well what may happen when meta-analytic research goes astray. It was concluded in a large meta-analysis of homoeopathic treatment that, overall, it had some effect (or as the authors put it: that their results were not compatible with the hypothesis that homoeopathy only has a placebo effect). In this case we know for sure that the treatment was ineffective (unless we believe that a drug can still be effective when it has been removed by repeated dilution) and therefore this study reveals the combined effect of different sources of bias both in the individual trials and in the combined analysis [132]. The meta-analysts faced the problem of publication bias (which they tried to tackle statistically), but they included studies of a large variety of very different clinical problems, and they admitted that two-thirds of the included trials were methodologically poor. Like others, they found that the higher the quality, the smaller the effect [154,155].

However, in the majority of cases there is no reason to question the result of a meta-analysis: the individual trials are comparable, their methodological standard is acceptable, and the meta-analysis is sufficiently thorough. In retrospect, there can be no doubt that meta-analyses could have saved many lives, if they had been done at the proper time. Streptokinase of acute myocardial infarction, for instance, could have been introduced 10–15 years earlier, if the community of cardiologists had been able to take a comprehensive view of the available evidence [156]. The same applies to corticosteroid treatment in imminent, premature labour [157]. In other cases ineffective or harmful treatments could have been abandoned if meta-analytic evidence had been available.

Meta-analyses also play an important role in clinical research. There are many examples of trials being repeated again and again in spite of the fact that the problem has already found its solution. Some of these unnecessary trials may have been done for commercial purposes, but sometimes the clinical investigators were simply unaware of the previous studies. Therefore, it ought to be an indispensable requirement that the protocol for a randomized trial contains a systematic review of those trials which have already been done.

From trials to clinical practice

The decisions taken in everyday clinical work must to the greatest possible extent be based on the results of clinical research. *Ideally, no treatment should be prescribed unless it has been demonstrated by randomized clinical trials, and preferably by meta-analyses, that it has the desired effect.*

Admittedly, there are exceptions to this rule as sometimes the effect is so obvious that it would be unreasonable to doubt uncontrolled experience. That was the case when ingestion of raw liver was introduced for the treatment of pernicious anaemia; previously all patients died, and now a complete cure was achieved. Those physicians who first used penicillin in acute streptococcal and pneumococcal infections were also quickly convinced of the efficiency of the new treatment, as were those who saw the first cures of childhood leukaemia and malignant seminomas. These are but a few accounts of unquestionable therapeutic breakthroughs, and, hopefully, there are more to come. When, for instance, some day in the future, we see the first cures for AIDS or for gastric cancer with liver metastases, we shall be convinced of the efficiency of the new treatment even without the evidence from randomized trials.

Such examples, however, are the exceptions rather than the rule. The effect of penicillin in some acute infections could not be questioned, but it is a very different matter to prove that a new antibiotic is superior to the existing ones, that some new cancer chemotherapy improves the patients' prognosis, or that a new antirheumatic drug is more powerful and has fewer side-effects than those already on the market. The breakthroughs are rare and far between, and in the vast majority of cases progress in therapy means the introduction of new treatments which are only a little better than those in current use, and under those circumstances the evidence from randomized trials is indispensable. We usually have great hopes when we decide to test a new treatment by doing a randomized trial, but experience shows that, on average, the new treatments which are tested in that way are no better, or only marginally better, than the ones with which they are compared [150,158–161].

Therefore, the need for randomized trials cannot be questioned, but it must be realized that the concept of fully evidence-based clinical practice remains an ideal which can never be attained. Firstly, some diseases or conditions are so rare that it is impossible, even in multicentre trials, to collect a sufficient number of patients. Secondly, the treatment response often depends on the stage and manifestations of the disease, and it is impossible to test all new treatments in every subgroup of patients presenting a particular clinical picture. Thirdly, there are situations where randomization may not be acceptable. Somebody who wishes to compare breast feeding and feeding with an artificial milk product will soon realize that most mothers will refuse random allocation.

It is also difficult to do therapeutic trials in malignant diseases which today are always fatal. Many patients will not accept the risk of being allocated to the control group, as they cling to the hope that the new treatment is effective and are willing to run the risk of unknown side-effects. This is a serious dilemma as, on one hand, it requires little empathy to understand this attitude, and, on the other, we must guard future patients against the introduction of new treatments that are ineffective or harmful. The situation is somewhat easier when some other treatment is available. Then it is possible to explain to the patients that it is necessary to do a comparative trial, testing the new treatment against the old one.

However, in spite of these difficulties we could get much closer to the ideal of evidence-based clinical practice than we are today. Most randomized trials are concerned with drug therapy, but new methods of physiotherapy and even recommendations about changes in lifestyle should also be tested rigorously. Some new surgical techniques have been subjected to randomized trials, but that is the exception and not the rule. Laparoscopic surgery is just one example of a therapeutic method which has become very popular in spite of the fact that in some conditions we lack good evidence of its superiority, and in Denmark the untimely introduction of a new type of cement (Boneloc) to be used in connection with hip replacements developed into a public scandal. This new product seemed very promising and very quickly it was accepted at departments of orthopaedic surgery both at home and abroad, until it was noted that in many cases the cement started to crumble a few years later. Probably, this complication could not have been predicted, but the number of patients who had to undergo a second operation would have been very much smaller if the use of the cement from the start had been confined to a properly conducted randomized trial.

We could also do better in the case of drug trials. In many countries it is impossible to register a new drug if it has not been tested by means of randomized clinical trials and the standard of clinical research has improved over the years, but readers of medical journals still frequently come across reports of trials that are much too small to provide reliable results or which are methodologically flawed in one way or another. In addition, there is a great need for many more meta-analyses, but the international Cochrane Collaboration is doing its best to remedy the situation in this respect.

It is also necessary to point out that contemporary clinical research, to an increasing extent, is biased by commercial interests. Clinical research ought to be inspired by those problems which clinicians encounter in their daily work, i.e. by those situations where they have to make a decision in spite of the fact that they do not really know what is best for the patient. Such situations occur frequently: is thrombolytic treatment warranted in this case of thrombophlebitis and pulmonary embolism, or is treatment with heparin and peroral anticoagulants better? And is it advisable to start life-long anticoagulant therapy, if the thrombophlebitis recurs? Is it necessary to give this patient penicillin intravenously? We have a shortage of staff, and could we not just as well use penicillin tablets? What is the best treatment of 'restless legs'. Does quinine have any effect at all? A survey of the literature will show that some randomized trials have been done addressing these and similar questions, but they are very few and far between compared with the number of trials testing different antirheumatic drugs, different H_2-antagonists and proton pump inhibitors against peptic ulcer, and β-blockers in a variety of diseases. The reason is, of course, that peroral anticoagulants, penicillin tablets and quinine have little commercial interest while the introduction, for instance, of a new antirheumatic drug may be associated with great profits. Such considerations ought to be quite irrelevant in public health services like those in the UK and the Nordic countries, but today economic constraints make it impossible to do large randomized trials without financial support from external sources.

It is also a big problem that more and more patients refuse to take part in randomized trials. Participation in any trial involves a certain degree of altruism, as the patients are well aware that they themselves may not benefit from the results. This reluctance may reflect the rise of individualism in modern society, but the commercialization may also play a role. Altruistic feelings will not induce patients to participate if they feel that the trial is motivated by commercial interests rather than the needs of future patients.

Clinical research workers may counteract this development by regarding their patients, not as objects of research, but as partners in the project. All patients who take part in a randomized trial ought to receive a letter after the conclusion of the project telling them which treatment they received and what the trial showed. That is very rarely done.

Treatment of the individual patient

This presentation might evoke the picture of the clinician sitting in front of his computer, entering the patient's clinical data, and then reading on the screen which treatment to give. It would of course be very helpful for the continued education of all medical practitioners if it became possible to link diagnoses, treatments and the results of meta-analyses in the databases, but there would still be a need for individualized clinical judgement. There will always be those cases where the diagnosis is not quite certain, those where the clinical picture is atypical and those where the patient suffers from two or more diseases and where the usual treatments for each of these cannot be combined.

As pointed out in connection with the diagnostic decision process (p. 87) it is no simple matter to use the experience gained from groups of patients for making decisions in the individual case. Clinical trials provide information about the statistical probability, i.e. the frequency of cure in a predefined population, whereas the clinician wishes to assess the (subjective) probability of cure in an individual patient. A randomized clinical trial may have shown that one treatment cured 20% more patients than another treatment, but this result only indicates that on average the chance of cure was 20% higher in one treatment group than in the other. Usually, the clinician acts on the assumption that his patient will respond as the average patient, but sometimes that is not reasonable. The comparison of a medical and a surgical treatment may have shown that surgery gave the best results, but the clinician who is faced with an elderly, frail patient may well judge that medical treatment will give his patient the best chances. The patient's own wishes may also influence the decision. Some people are frightened by the very idea of a surgical operation and then it might also be advisable to prefer medical treatment.

Often the clinician has the choice between different medical treatments, which have all proved effective in randomized trials, but which have never been compared with one another. Here economic considerations may determine the choice, both for the patient's sake and for the sake of society. Usually, new drugs are more expensive than those already on the market, *and they should not be prescribed unless it has been shown by randomized trials, and preferably by a meta-analysis, that they are better than the old ones.* Unfortunately, there are numerous examples where effective marketing made doctors disregard this principle. New synthetic opiates have been accepted as, allegedly, the risk of addiction was smaller, and new antirheumatic drugs have been preferred to the old ones because they were said to be more powerful and less ulcerogenic, but in these and many other cases it was found later that the assertions were false.

Clinicians in their attempts to keep up-to-date should only rely on un-biased sources, and as a general rule they should pay no attention to information from advertisements and representatives from drug firms. One would never expect a car dealer to admit that his cars are more expensive, but no better, than those of the competitors, and, similarly, a doctor cannot possibly expect to be told by the agent of a pharmaceutical company that there is no reliable evidence that his new drug is better than other, cheaper ones already on the market. This is not a criticism of the drug firms who only pursue their legitimate commercial interests, but a criticism of the naivety of many doctors.

CHAPTER 7

Medicine and the Humanities

Surely there exists no wider gulf, nor more stubborn resistance to bridging it, than that which for centuries has separated science and humanities in medicine. That this should be so in medicine is a remarkable paradox, for medicine, after all, is by its very nature a human science, historically perhaps the very first human science. [Engel [162]]

There is a strong tendency to-day to identify knowledge with natural science. But, as two wars have made us painfully aware, natural science can only tell us the means, not how these means ought to be used . . . The study of science must therefore be supplemented by a study of the right way of using the knowledge it provides. [Ewing [163]]

The four components of clinical reasoning

Traditionally, a distinction is made between science and the humanities. Natural scientists are observers of nature, whereas their counterparts from the humanities take an interest in human feelings and endeavour to understand and interpret all the different ways in which human beings express themselves. Scientists seek the causes of the phenomena they observe and try to establish the laws of nature, whereas humanists, as we shall call them, are concerned with reasons rather than causes [25].

It is one of the fascinations of clinical medicine that it belongs to both these two worlds. The clinician uses the scientific approach when she regards her patient's disease as an objective phenomenon to be observed, explained and perhaps remedied, but at the same time she adopts a humanistic approach seeing her patient as a human being whose situation she must try to understand. This chapter deals with the humanistic approach, but before we proceed to that topic we shall take a comprehensive view of the structure of clinical reasoning (Table 12).

Table 12 The four components of the basis of clinical decisions.

Scientific thinking
1   *The deductive component*
Inferences from theoretical knowledge about diseases and disease mechanisms
2   *The empirical component*
Inferences from experience gained from the study of previous patients
Uncontrolled experience
Controlled experience
Humanistic thinking
3   *The empathic–hermeneutic component*
Inferences from an understanding of the patient as a fellow human being
4   *The ethical component*
Inferences from ethical norms

In the preceding parts of this book we have tried to analyse clinical thinking from a scientific point of view and we have pointed out that scientific reasoning has two components. Firstly, the decision about the diagnosis or the decision to institute a particular treatment may be the result of theoretical considerations. This means that the clinician tries to deduce from her theoretical knowledge of the structure and functions of the human organism what is the patient's diagnosis and what treatment will have the desired effect. This is the deductive component of scientific reasoning. Secondly, the diagnostic or therapeutic decision may be based on experience, i.e. uncontrolled or controlled experience which was gained in the past by the examination or treatment of similar patients. This is the empirical component of scientific reasoning.

We shall not repeat the discussion of the relative merits of these types of reasoning, but only recapitulate that deductions from theoretical knowledge can rarely be trusted due to the complexity of the functions of the human organism, and that, for a number of reasons, uncontrolled experience is also unreliable (Chapter 5). Therefore, our decisions must as far as possible be based on controlled experience, especially studies of the value of diagnostic tests, using the direct method (Chapter 4), and randomized clinical trials (Chapter 6).

In this chapter we shall focus on the humanistic approach to clinical decision-making which also has two components, which we shall label the empathic–hermeneutic component and the ethical component.

The empathic–hermeneutic component

Disease or illness, according to the humanistic approach, is the way in which the individual patient experiences and interprets the different symptoms in the context of her own life. This experience is often associated with anxiety and suffering, and the clinical decision-maker must try to understand what the patient really feels. Therefore empathy, which is the ability to see oneself in somebody else's situation, is an important clinical concept.

In some cases empathic understanding is quite straightforward. Consider, for instance, a male middle-aged consultant who in the out-patient department sees a male, middle-aged academic who lives in the same part of the town. Then doctor and patient have much the same background, and, probably, they will find it very easy to understand each other.

But perhaps the next patient seen by this consultant is a young female immigrant from Turkey who tells him about her problems. There is no language problem at all as her English is fluent, but empathy fails as the consultant knows too little about her background to be able to see the situation from her point of view. If he had had Turkish friends or had spent some time in a Turkish village, or if he had just read some books about Turkish family life, he would have been in a better position. The point is that empathy requires knowledge, and it was lacking in this case. This knowledge, which is needed to understand another person from that person's perspective, is called *hermeneutic knowledge* (from Greek *hermeneutike* = art of interpretation).

Empathy, however, may fail for other reasons than lack of knowledge about a patient's cultural background. Few doctors, for instance, have experienced what it means to receive a diagnosis of incurable cancer, or to be admitted to hospital due to sudden and unexpected praecordial pain, and very few have tried to live their lives as dialysis patients or to have a permanent ileostomy. Doctors who see many such patients may gradually acquire the necessary hermeneutic knowledge, but there is a shortcut which is not sufficiently appreciated. Knowledge, including hermeneutic knowledge, can be committed to writing and communicated to others. We remember a colleague who, like many others, found it difficult to talk to incurably ill cancer patients. He felt that these patients, who had been told that they would die within a limited period of time, were living in a world of their own which he could not penetrate. Then he read Kübler-Ross' book '*On Death and Dying*' [164] which reports what this author learnt by interviewing 200 incurable cancer patients at regular intervals. She quotes what the patients told her, often using their own words, and she describes the stages of denial, anger, bargaining, depression and, finally, acceptance. After having spent a few hours reading this small book, the colleague found it much easier to understand his patients, e.g. the patient who seemed to have 'forgotten' what she had been told about her prognosis and was now busy planning her life several years ahead, the patient who during previous visits had been very composed, but now met everybody with anger and accusations, and the patient who said that she was willing to die if only once more, sitting in her garden, she could experience the coming of spring.

Kübler-Ross' book may be regarded as an early example of a *qualitative* study or, as it ought to be called, a *hermeneutic* study, and we shall illustrate this kind of research by two other examples. A Danish doctor interviewed a number of patients who had made an appointment with their general practitioner and, after the visits had taken place, she interviewed the doctors and repeated the interviews of the patients [165]. The general impression was a positive one, of patients trusting their doctors and of doctors trying to understand their patients, but the communication between them was by no means perfect. The general practitioners often thought that they were expected to write a prescription when, in fact, the patients' primary wish was not treatment, but just an explanation of their symptoms.

Doctors, of course, provide such explanations, but when they do, they tend to talk about anatomical lesions and physiological malfunction and that does not satisfy the patients who search for the cause in their daily lives. Many misunderstandings could be avoided if doctors, at the beginning of each consultation, spent a little more time letting their patients talk freely about their illness, the way the symptoms affect their daily lives, their fears for the future and what they themselves believe caused the illness. It is important that the history is as complete as possible, but too much essential information is lost if the questioning is reduced to a series of brief questions (Where does it hurt? Did the pain radiate? In what direction?). The scientific approach invites the systematic collection of well-defined data, whereas the humanistic approach requires that the patient's illness is seen in the context of the patient's life.

The interest in hermeneutic research is on the increase, especially among nurses, but unfortunately the results are rarely published in the ordinary medical journals. One study, done by a Danish nurse, focussed on patients with chronic renal disease [166]. She interviewed patients receiving haemodialysis either in hospital or in their own homes, patients waiting for a donor kidney, patients who had received one, and patients who had suffered rejection of the graft. These categories of patients experienced their situation very differently, and the study communicates essential hermeneutic knowledge which it may take years to acquire, working at a nephrology unit.

The methods used in such studies were first developed by anthropologists and sociologists [167]. They differ from conventional scientific ones in a number of respects, e.g. the selection of patients, the choice of interview technique and the analysis of the results, but they also require meticulous planning, a detailed protocol and stringent reasoning.

The ethical component

Scientific reasoning guided by empathic understanding is an essential part of clinical decision-making, but it has its limitations. Scientists can answer questions like these: 'What *is* the patient's diagnosis?', 'What *can* we do?' or 'What *are* the outcomes of these treatments in this randomized trial?, but they cannot tell us what we *ought* to do in a particular situation. It is impossible to make this jump from the 'is' and the 'can' of the world of science and technology to the 'ought' of clinical practice without including a value judgement. We must decide whether the consequences of our actions are good or bad and whether the actions themselves are acceptable, and such value judgements belong to the sphere of ethics. Therefore, clinical decision-making always has an ethical component.

Very often the value judgement which determines the decision is so uncontroversial that it is not noted. It is, for instance, a fact that most patients who have developed a cataract and are almost blind will regain their faculty of vision when the lens is removed, and it is tempting to conclude from this statement that therefore we ought to remove the lens in patients with this disease, but this conclusion cannot be deduced from the facts alone. It also depends on the value judgement that it is better to see than to be blind. If we make the absurd assumption that the opposite were true, it would of course be wrong to do this operation.

In other cases the situation is less simple. There are, for instance, three different treatments of hyperthyroidism, the popularity of which has varied over the years: long-term treatment with antithyroid drugs; subtotal thyroidectomy; and treatment with radioactive iodine. The decision how to treat these patients depends among other things on their age, the size of the goitre and the possibility of pregnancy, and, obviously, we must pay great attention to the results of follow-up studies, preferably in the form of randomized trials. These trials, however, do not provide the final answer. We must also make complex value judgements balancing the risk of post-operative vocal cord paralysis against the possible side-effects of antithyroid drugs and the possibility of myxoedema following treatment with radioactive iodine. These values cannot be determined once and for all, as they depend on the preferences of the individual patient.

Some doctors seem to hold the view that clinical medicine is a scientific discipline, and that medical ethics are no more than a set of rules which must be respected when we are dealing with patients. They have missed the point which was first made by the philosopher David Hume: you can never derive an 'ought' from an 'is'. All clinical decisions require value judgements and the ethical component must never be overlooked.

Three kinds of norms

Ethics and morality* concern what we ought to do and what is good, but it is worth noticing that these (and similar) normative words are also used in non-ethical (non-moral) contexts. Confusion arises when we overlook the distinction between technical, legal and ethical norms.

Technical norms tell us what is good, or effective, for reaching certain pre-defined goals, regardless of the moral goodness of those goals. Thus, a good knife is a sharp knife, and a good revolver is one which makes you hit the bull's eye. Defiance of technical norms is an invitation to practical difficulties as we may not, for instance, be able to cut what we want to cut with a blunt knife, or to hit what we want to hit with a bad revolver. Technical norms are established by means of scientific methods and in many contexts they may also be termed scientific norms. A good or effective antihypertensive drug is one which, according to the results of randomized trials, lowers the blood pressure, but it is quite possible that the lowering of the blood pressure reduces the patient's quality of life.

Legal norms determine what we may do and may not do according to the law, and if we defy those norms we may be punished. A gynaecologist may feel that it is morally justified to do an abortion, but, if it is illegal in that situation, she may run into serious trouble.

Ethical or moral norms differ from the other two types as they tell us which actions and which consequences are good in themselves (intrinsically good), and those who violate these norms will be met with the moral indignation of others or suffer a guilty conscience. Different people may accept different norms, but most of us agree that it is intrinsically good to speak the truth and to help other people, and that pain and suffering are intrinsically bad. If we state that we ought to institute a certain treatment in order to ensure the patient a good quality of life, we are also using the word good in its ethical sense as a person's quality of life is good or bad in itself.

---

* We use the words *ethical* and *moral* (as well as *ethics* and *moral* philosophy) synonymously, which is defensible from an etymological point of view, as Greek *ethos* and Latin *mores* orginally had the same meaning (habits or customs).

It is important not to mix up these three kinds of norms, although it is easy to do so as the same statement may sometimes be interpreted in different ways. The sentence: 'You ought not give this young girl those contraceptive pills' may refer to a legal norm (i.e. it is forbidden to do so, according to the law, without the parents' consent), a technical norm (i.e. scientific studies have shown that these pills cause more adverse effects than other pills) or an ethical norm (i.e. if you do it you are acting immorally).

Medical doctors sometimes find it difficult to distinguish between scientific (technical) and ethical norms. A transplantation surgeon, for instance, once said that there was no ethical problem if he had only one organ at his disposal, but two patients who needed one. He would just give the organ to that patient who would be ensured the best prognosis. Consequently, if he had had two female patients, one who was childless and one who had two children, he would presumably have disregarded that fact, but by doing so he would have taken the ethical stance that being responsible for small children is ethically irrelevant.

Lawyers and some ethicists who focus on individual rights, on their part, tend not to distinguish too sharply between ethical and legal norms. It is often seen, especially in American literature on medical ethics, that ethical problems from clinical practice are reduced to a legal discussion of patients' rights.

The foundation of health care ethics

For a period of three months the doctors from the medical department of a large hospital were asked to make a note each time they faced a significant ethical problem, i.e. a situation where they were in doubt which decision to make or suspected that some of their colleagues might have decided differently. During those three months 426 patients were admitted to the department and in 25% of these cases the doctors recorded one or more such problems [168].

This example illustrates well the importance of ethical reasoning in clinical practice, and it is quite justified that medical ethics is now being recognized as an academic discipline in its own right. However, it is also important to realize that ethical norms vary in different parts of the world and that medical ethics must be taught differently in different countries. Medical ethics is not international as are the scientific medical disciplines. Admittedly, a number of international organizations have issued ethical declarations on a variety of medical topics, but they rarely offer much guidance in the concrete case. They may be helpful in the sense that they establish certain international guidelines at a time of increasing international co-operation, but at best they represent 'the smallest common denominator' for the norms in different societies, and at worst they are dominated by the norms of one particular culture.

This book is intended for an international readership, and therefore we shall stress the structure of ethical reasoning rather than the solution of the problems. We do not, however, wish to conceal our own ethical intuitions, and we shall describe openly the approach to health care ethics to which we have committed ourselves. It is, we believe, the approach which prevails in those European countries that have a public health service (such as the Nordic countries and the UK) and those which seek the same general goal by means of some sort of universal health insurance scheme. The ethical basis of the health services in these countries is best described by means of three principles:

1   *The Samaritan principle*, i.e. the obligation of all citizens to help each other in case of illness.

2   *The principle of distributive justice*, i.e. the obligation to ensure a just distribution of the limited resources of the health service.

3   *The principle of autonomy*, i.e. the obligation to respect the individual right to self-determination.

The Samaritan principle must be regarded as a fundamental ethical principle in our part of the world, as health services which offer free hospital treatment to everybody would make no sense if people did not accept this obligation. The principle stresses our mutual obligations and it may therefore be seen as a special case of the Golden Rule 'to do unto others as you would have them do unto you' [169]. This idea of reciprocity is recognized not only in the Christian tradition, but also by many other cultures and religions. In modern societies with a public health care system the individual citizens may be said to fulfil their Samaritan duty by paying for the health service which then employs professional Samaritans, i.e. doctors, nurses, etc., to carry out the Samaritan work.

The resources of any health service, however, are limited and therefore it is also necessary to accept a principle of distributive justice or, as it was once said, to ensure 'that everybody gets a fair share of the national health cake'. Thirdly, the countries in question are democratic, and therefore the Samaritan activities of the health service must be carried out in such a way that due respect is paid to individual autonomy.

None of these principles should be accepted at face value. The Golden Rule has many interpretations, the concept of justice is a controversial topic, and respect for autonomy, which we shall discuss below, has been understood differently by different philosophers. However, the principles provide a starting point for our ethical deliberations, and they reveal the difference between health care ethics in, for instance, Europe and the United States. American ethicists also formulate basic principles, but usually the principle of autonomy comes first, and the formulation of the Samaritan principle (which they call the principle of beneficence) is much weaker. Once it was stated in an ethical declaration that 'all persons have some moral obligation to benefit others, to some degree, perhaps especially those who are in need', and, according to that view, the goal of the public health care system is limited to ensuring 'universal access to an acceptable, decent minimum of basic health care' [170,171]. We do not, however, wish to draw too sharp a line between North American and European health care ethics. Libertarian norms, like the American ones, are gaining ground in Europe, the Canadian norms seem closer to those in Europe than those in the United States, and in the United States there are many people who see the need for health service reforms.

The structure of ethical reasoning

Some doctors seem to think that it is a futile exercise to discuss ethical problems, as in the last resort moral statements express no more than the feelings of the speaker. This view of ethics (which moral philosophers call *emotivism*) is fallacious, as ethical problems, just like scientific ones, can be subjected to a logical analysis. First of all, ethical reasoning must be consistent, which means that like cases must be treated alike, or, to put it differently, that a person who decides to do one thing in one situation and another thing in another situation must be able to state the ethically relevant difference. A doctor once argued that the moment of conception marks the beginning of a human life, that the wilful interruption of a human life is murder, and that, consequently, abortion amounts to murder; but this doctor also said that he accepted contraception by means of an intrauterine device. He obviously felt intuitively that the two situations differed, but he ought to have realized that his argument against abortion also applied to that form of contraception. If he had understood that ethical problems require logical reasoning, he would have considered the problem more closely.

It would also be most unfortunate if ethics committees, including those which review medical research, regarded ethics as a question of personal feelings. Their answers to ethical problems may not be true or false in any objective sense, but they must have subjected them to a thorough analysis. It is quite justified to accuse the members of an ethics committee of incompetence if they do not act consistently and are unable to justify their decisions rationally.

The ethical decision process is a stepwise procedure. The very first step is the recognition of the problem, and it cannot be taken for granted that all doctors are skilful in this respect. The project where the staff at a medical department were asked to record all significant ethical problems illustrated that it requires training. Prior to the study the doctors had had no particular interest in medical ethics and at the beginning they saw very few problems, but gradually they learnt to recognize the ethical component of their decisions. It is one of the most important goals of the teaching of medical ethics to undergraduates that they learn to detect those ethical problems which they are likely to face as medical practitioners, so that they do not, as the transplantation surgeon mentioned above, overlook the ethical component of their decisions.

The recognition of an ethical problem is tantamount to the recognition of a conflict between different ethical considerations, but usually we intuitively feel what is right and wrong and what would be the best decision. This initial intuition will reflect our own ethical norms, the norms of the society in which we live, as well as generally accepted professional norms. We can no longer say that the practice of medicine must be regarded as a vocation to help others, but the driving force behind all clinical decisions must still be the wish to relieve human suffering and to combine technical expertise with true compassion and understanding. The ethical and the empathic components of the clinical decision process cannot be separated. A wise clinician once recommended the use of the *uncle test*, by which he meant that the doctor should imagine that the patient was a dear uncle of hers. Whenever she faced an ethical problem, she should ask the following question: how would I like my uncle's doctor to act in this situation? The uncle test seems preferable to a spouse, child or parent test, as it ensures that the decision-maker has warm feelings, but is not so emotionally involved that she cannot think rationally.

However, the immediate intuition and the 'uncle test' will not provide adequate answers to complex ethical dilemmas. It is necessary to proceed with a rational analysis of the problem at hand, including both factual and ethical considerations.

Assessment of the facts of the case

When different people disagree about the answer to an ethical problem it will often be found that their ethical attitudes are much the same, but that their assessment of the facts differ. The factual basis of the problem must in this connection be interpreted very broadly, as it comprises not only the assessment of the clinical data and the patient's situation, but also the assessment of the prognosis and the probable outcome of different decisions. Imagine, for instance, the situation where one doctor recommends resuscitation of a patient who has suffered a stroke whereas a colleague finds that the patient should be allowed to die. It is possible that these colleagues have similar ethical norms, but that their assessment differed as regards the patient's condition, the likely prognosis after resuscitation and the wishes of the relatives.

Participants in ethical debates often appeal to the so-called slippery slope argument. They may find that some action is morally acceptable here and now, but hold that it should not be allowed, as they fear that it would lead to other practices which they regard as morally unacceptable. Some people, for example, argue that active euthanasia may be morally acceptable in some terminal cancer cases, but that it should not be legalized as it might lead to euthanasia in other situations where it is quite unacceptable. In such cases the assessment of the consequences, if they occur, is an ethical problem, but the assessment of the likelihood that they will occur is a factual problem.

Consequential considerations

Consequential considerations play a very important role in the ethical decision process. They serve to compare the 'goodness' of the consequences of different actions, and that is not always easy to do.

In our daily lives there are many situations where we have the choice between different decisions, and then we usually start by considering the consequences for particular individuals, especially members of our family, friends and colleagues. These are the *person-orientated* consequential considerations. Often, however, we must think further than that. We must, for instance, take into account the general consequences for other people if we do not pay our income tax as required or if we pollute the environment unnecessarily. In such cases it is tempting to make the excuse that the consequences of one's own action are insignificant in a larger perspective, but then one may generalize the consequential consideration and ask: what would the general consequences be if everybody acted that way under similar circumstances? This question serves as a guide to the *universal* consequential considerations.

The ethics of the doctor–patient relationship can be described in much the same way. The clinician sees it as her primary goal to do the best for her patient and, if she has the choice between different actions, she must try to decide which one is likely to have the best consequences in that particular case. These patient-orientated consequential considerations may be quite complicated as they require not only that she compares the goodness of all possible outcomes, but also that she assesses the probability that these outcomes will occur. A very good consequence (curing the patient) may counterbalance a very bad consequence (a serious complication) if the probability of the former is sufficiently high and that of the latter sufficiently small. The assessment of the goodness of a consequence is a value judgement and as such it belongs to the realm of ethics, whereas the assessment of the probability requires empirical evidence and belongs to the realm of science.

Statistical decision theorists [6] have suggested that these consequential considerations may be formalized by 'measuring' the goodness or utility (U) of the different consequences on an interval scale from 0 to 1. Then, if we know the probability of these consequences, it becomes possible to calculate the expected utility, $\Sigma(P \times U)$, of each decision, i.e. the average 'amount of goodness' produced by that decision. This procedure illustrates well the logic of consequential considerations, but obviously it cannot be used in practice. The goodness of a consequence for a particular person cannot be measured in centimetres or any other interval scale.

Other person-orientated considerations may also be needed as the clinician may have to assess the consequences for the patient's relatives and sometimes also the consequences for herself. Apart from that, universal considerations may be required to assess the consequences for the health service and for future patients. We shall illustrate the complexity of these consequential considerations by means of some examples, but first we shall consider a very different type of ethical consideration.

Deontological considerations

Some moral philosophers who call themselves utilitarians or consequentialists hold that ethical reasoning is no more than an assessment of consequences, but we believe that most people would deny that. They would not accept that the end always justifies the means, as they believe that some actions, regardless of the consequences, are more acceptable than others from an ethical point of view.

Therefore, it is necessary to take into account a very different type of ethical consideration, which is usually called *deontological* (from Greek *deon* = duty) although it does not only concern our duties, but also our rights. The deontological way of thinking is well illustrated by the Ten Commandments in the Old Testament. One of the commandments reads: Thou shalt not steal! It does not say that it is forbidden, if the consequences are bad, but that it is quite permissible if (as in the case of Robin Hood) the consequences are good. It is the act of stealing as such that is objectionable from a moral point of view.

The most important deontological principles in medical ethics are the duties to respect the patient's autonomy, to preserve life, to speak the truth, to respect the patient's dignity and to maintain confidentiality. All these duties are important, but in spite of that we must realize that it is difficult to imagine a deontological principle which is absolute. Life must be preserved by active treatment, except when the quality of that life is very low, and the maintenance of confidentiality is essential, except for those rare cases where the interests of society or other individuals must take priority. Therefore, moral duties are said to be *prima facie* duties, which means that they are morally binding except in those cases where other (deontological or consequential) considerations have greater weight.

The ethical decision

Finally, the clinical decision-maker must decide which action is the most acceptable one from an ethical point of view, and in some cases the different kinds of considerations have clarified the situation to such an extent that she is in no doubt what to do. In other cases, however, the dilemma is not solved that easily. The clinician feels that she has taken into account all the important consequential and deontological considerations and she realizes that, on balance, they call for one particular decision, but unfortunately she also feels that she cannot reconcile that conclusion with her ethical intuition and basic ethical beliefs. In that case she can do no more than rethink the problem once again and search her mind for those ethical considerations which determined her intuition, and if she finds none, she may well experience that during the analytic process her intuition gradually changes. However, ethical dilemmas do not always have an unequivocal solution. Experienced clinicians, facing a difficult decision, sometimes know in advance that, whatever they do, they will be left with a guilty conscience.

We do not suggest, of course, that the clinician should always sit down and make a list of all the different consequential and deontological considerations, although sometimes it might not be a bad idea. Most of the ethical problems which medical practitioners face in ordinary clinical practice are not unique, and they will have adopted a policy of their own, as regards, for example, the information of cancer patients or the treatment of those who are terminally ill. Routine, however, should never prevail to such an extent that they forget that they are faced with an ethical problem and that each patient is unique.

It is also important, especially at hospitals in a public health service, that clinical decisions do not depend too much on the ethical norms of one particular doctor. Patients rarely choose their doctors themselves, and even when they do, they cannot know very much about their ethical policies. Therefore, before they make the decisions, doctors ought to discuss all major ethical problems, both with their colleagues and with those nurses who know the patient well. Such conferences may reveal that the doctor presenting a problem has overlooked some important ethical consideration, and in the long run the discussions will promote a harmonization of the ethical norms at that particular department.

Quality of life

The most important consequential considerations are, of course, the patient-orientated ones which aim at choosing that decision which has the best consequences for the patient. The meaning of the word 'best' in this context is uncontroversial if it is simply a question of curing the patient or of removing unpleasant symptoms, but in other contexts it is not so simple to decide what is good and what is not so good, and it is in such cases that it has become fashionable to talk about quality of life.

The expression quality of life is used in different ways, and it is never defined in exact terms. Most often, it denotes something subjective, and in that sense it is used in much the same way as decision theorists use the word utility and moral philosophers, about two hundred years ago, talked about happiness. At that time the utilitarian philosopher, Jeremy Bentham, tried to develop what he called a felicific calculus in order to measure happiness, and that idea, which later was completely abandoned by moral philosophers, has now been revived by those who believe that it is possible to measure the utility of different decisions or the patients' subjective quality of life on some interval scale. We shall not discuss the methods which have been suggested, as none of them are practicable.

In a medical context we face the additional conceptual problem that we should not concern ourselves with the patient's subjective quality of life as such, but only with her health-related quality of life. It is a medical problem if the reduction of a patient's quality of life is caused by her illness, but not, if it is caused by family trouble or problems at work.

Quality of life is also sometimes used in an objective sense as something which can be observed, and within limits that is a reasonable idea. Human beings may differ but presumably we should all feel that our subjective quality of life was reduced if arthritic changes made it difficult for us to climb stairs, dress or take a bath, or if a cataract prevented us from reading the morning paper or looking at TV. Therefore, it is very important both in everyday clinical practice and for research purposes that all such disabilities are recorded and perhaps quantified by means of simple rating scales, but it is much less obvious that it should be possible to combine the observations and to calculate some sort of objective quality of life score. Usually, the weighting of the individual items is quite arbitrary, and the validity of the resulting score remains a matter of belief.

Thus, quality of life measurements remain a dubious affair, but we should of course listen to our patients when they tell us about their lives and we should try to take a comprehensive view of their clinical condition. Such informal judgements play an important role in the decision process, and sometimes we find that there is little agreement between the quality of life as it is experienced by the patient herself and our assessment of the patient's quality of life. We see some patients who appear to be in a very poor state, but still claim that they are very happy. They seem to have reduced their expectations of life and to have accepted their condition. Others complain that their lives are completely ruined by some symptom or disability which from the doctor's point of view seems rather trivial. They seem to have expected a life devoid of health problems of any kind.

Up to now we have only considered the quality of life at a given moment in time, but clinicians also wish to predict their patient's condition in the years to come. Decision theorists have tried to formalize such predictions, and their approach has provoked considerable debate. They suggest that doctors should calculate the number of quality-adjusted life years or QALYs, i.e. the number of years that a patient is expected to live multiplied by her quality of life (measured on a scale from 0 to 1). This product is thought to represent the 'amount of quality of life' which the patient is expected to accumulate during the remaining part of her life. If different treatments are available, one should calculate the number of QALYs which is produced by each of these, and then choose the one which from this point of view ensures the best prognosis. We have already mentioned that it is impossible to measure quality of life on an interval scale, but apart from that the idea is conceptually bizarre as it is assumed that it is as good to live one year with a quality of life of 1 as to live 10 years with a quality of life of 0.1.

Nevertheless, it is important that clinicians take an interest in the age-old concept of 'a good life'. Nowadays few people die young from acute infections or accidents, and it is necessary to discuss how we wish our lives to end. The majority will probably say that they would like to keep fit and live to a great age (without specifying what they mean by that) and then die suddenly. They fear above anything else that they will grow senile and helpless, so that they have to spend the last part of their life in a nursing home. We often say, when somebody dies whom we knew well, that this person had a good life except for the last few years which she would have been better without. Epidemiologists regularly report that a large number of sudden deaths from myocardial infarction, mostly among elderly people, could have been prevented if people changed their lifestyle in one way or another, and their findings are widely publicized through the media. They forget to tell us that some of these sudden deaths forestalled an end to life which very few people would wish for themselves.

Autonomy and paternalism

Autonomy and paternalism are key concepts in medical ethics. An *autonomous decision* is a decision which is made after due consideration without external coercion, and an *autonomous person* is a person who is able to make such decisions. In contrast, a non-autonomous or incompetent person is someone who for some reason or other is unable to do so. We have already mentioned the principle of autonomy, which for all practical purposes is interpreted as the duty to respect the individual's right to self-determination.

Moral philosophers use different definitions of *paternalism*, but here we shall say that a person *A* acts paternalistically towards another person *B*, when *A*—with or without *B*'s consent—chooses that decision which she believes has the best consequences for *B*. Using this definition, a distinction may be made between three forms of paternalism: genuine, solicited and unsolicited paternalism.

Genuine paternalism is paternalistic action towards non-autonomous persons, and the typical example is the father (*pater*) who imposes his will on his small child 'because daddy knows best'. But it is not only children who must be regarded as non-autonomous. Doctors see patients who are unconscious, delirious because of a high temperature, psychotic or severely mentally handicapped, and in all such cases there is no doubt that paternalistic action is morally required.

Solicited paternalism is paternalistic action towards autonomous patients who have said that they have no wish to take part in the decision process but wish to leave the decisions to the doctor. If the wish has been expressed unambiguously, this type of paternalism is also morally acceptable.

Unsolicited paternalism is paternalistic action towards autonomous patients without their consent, i.e. those situations where a doctor institutes diagnostic procedures or treatments without having consulted the patient in advance. Doctors should of course always make up their mind which decisions will serve their patients' interests best, but that does not necessarily imply that those decisions should be implemented. To use the terminology which was introduced above, the patient-orientated consequential considerations are subject to the deontological constraint that the patient's autonomy must be respected. Today it is agreed, at least in this part of the world, that as a general rule unsolicited paternalism is morally unacceptable.

There can be little doubt that previously most doctors indulged much too much in unsolicited paternalism, and that today the great majority of patients expect that their autonomy is respected. However, it must also be realized that there is no sharp distinction between autonomy and non-autonomy, and that, consequently, there is a grey zone between genuine and unsolicited paternalism. Paediatricians must take into account the degree of maturity of the individual child, psychiatrists face particularly difficult ethical and legal problems when they consider treatment against the patient's own wish, and all other clinicians see numerous borderline cases where it is a matter of judgement whether or not paternalistic action is justified.

In some cases one may even talk about a selective loss of autonomy. Many drug addicts must be regarded as fully autonomous in many respects but, due to their physical dependence on the drugs, those actions which are related to the abuse cannot be regarded as autonomous. Their right to self-determination must be respected in many situations, but genuine paternalism may be required when the decisions concern the addictive behaviour. Therapists sometimes talk about establishing 'contracts' with addicts, and that may be reasonable from a pedagogical point of view, but these contracts do not have the same moral status as ordinary contracts between autonomous persons.

It is impossible in this book to cover all aspects of clinical ethics, but we have selected a number of illustrative examples. The discussion of these cases is only meant to illustrate important aspects of the structure of ethical reasoning. Thus, we do not seek to promote any particular ethical views, although we shall not try to conceal our own ethical attitudes.

Clinical examples

Example 1

A 55-year-old woman has felt a dull pain below the right costal margin and is referred to hospital by her general practitioner. Ultrasonically guided biopsies revealed metastases from an adenocarcinoma in both liver lobes. It is concluded that there is no effective treatment. What should the patient be told? This example will be used to illustrate some important aspects of ethical reasoning. The considerations vary from case to case, but as a starting point it is often useful to ask the following three questions:

1   Which decision will have the best consequences for my patient? This is the patient-orientated consequential consideration mentioned above, and it is related to the Samaritan principle of health care ethics.

2   What would the general consequences be if all doctors acted in that way under similar circumstances? This is the universal consequential consideration, and one of the examples below will illustrate the connection between this question and the principle of justice.

3   Is my patient autonomous, and, if so, do I respect my patient's right to self-determination? This is a deontological consideration which corresponds to the principle of autonomy.

As regards the first of these questions, most doctors would probably say that in this case it is best for the patient to be informed about the diagnosis and prognosis. They will argue that in the long run it will not be possible to conceal the diagnosis from her, and that it will be much easier to support her if she is told the truth from the start. Apart from that there may be many things of a practical nature which she would wish to settle while there is still time.

Then, according to the second question, we should ask ourselves what would happen if all doctors concealed the diagnosis from cancer patients, and again we must conclude that, in general, patients ought to be told the truth. When patients, as in this case, are going to die from their disease, the diagnosis will be revealed sooner or later, and it would become general knowledge that doctors lie. That might cause lack of trust in the medical profession, and it might have the secondary effect that patients with chronic benign diseases suffered unnecessarily. They would not believe the doctor who told them quite truthfully that their disease was not malignant. Further, we must consider those patients who are cured from their cancer, e.g. patients with a colonic cancer who are cured by a colonic resection. If they were never told that they had had a cancer, people would only hear about those cancer patients who died, and the population would be led to believe that cancer is always incurable. These considerations are not theoretical, as we experienced these effects when doctors, only three or four decades ago, rarely told their patients the true diagnosis.

The answer to the third question points in the same direction. Withholding the information would be a violation of the patient's autonomy, as the patient cannot decide what to do with the limited rest of her life if she is not adequately informed.

We are aware of the fact that some readers will disagree with our answers to the three questions. A large international survey has shown that almost all Northern European and North American doctors would tell such a patient the truth, but that most doctors in Southern Europe and especially Eastern Europe would conceal the diagnosis and prognosis [172]. This difference must reflect differences as regards both ethical norms and factual beliefs. Obviously, doctors in Southern and Eastern Europe do not stress the third deontological consideration as much as their Northern European colleagues do today, but they must also believe, as Northern European doctors did a few decades ago, that telling the truth would cause greater psychological distress. This survey also showed that Southern and Eastern European doctors always told the spouse the full truth, for which reason their information policy will not have all those general effects which were recorded as the answer to the second question.

Obviously, the policy of openness does not imply that patients should just be told the crude facts. The information must be part of a dialogue where the clinician feels her way, notices the patient's reaction, finds out how much the patient wishes to know at that particular moment, and offers further consultations. In other words, adequate information presupposes empathic understanding. When, for instance, the doctor uses the word cancer, she must be aware of the fact that it will be interpreted very differently by different patients. One patient may have known somebody who was completely cured while somebody else may have witnessed one of those tragic cases where the disease was particularly protracted and painful.

Example 2

An 84-year-old man is referred to hospital because of a slight anginal pain, and a chest X-ray reveals a shadow which, probably, is caused by a cancer that as yet has produced no symptoms. The patient's general condition precludes surgical intervention. What should this patient be told?

Most doctors who are told about this case seem to agree that it was unfortunate that this somewhat unnecessary X-ray picture was ever taken, implying that it would be best for the patient to remain ignorant of this finding. But that which is best is not always right and some colleagues have argued that the principle of autonomy must be upheld and that the patient must be told.

This is a real case and the clinician in charge applied the uncle test (p. 156). She argued that her imaginary, very sensible 84-year-old uncle would be well aware of the fact that he would not live forever. He would by that time have drawn up a will (if he wanted to make one) and he enjoyed each day. Why should one pester the life of the dear old uncle with this information? She also argued (not quite convincingly) that withholding the information was not a violation of autonomy, but an example of what she called 'implicit solicited paternalism', as she was sure that the old man would not have wanted the information, if one had asked him. As a result of these considerations the patient was not told anything, but the clinician did inform the patient's general practitioner that she had seen a lesion in the lung which might be a cancer.

We feel that it would be more honest to say that this was a clearcut example of unsolicited paternalism, where the clinician felt that the patient-orientated consequential consideration took priority over the duty to respect the patient's autonomy. But we have to admit that we sympathize with this colleague who acted out of true compassion. Respect for autonomy requires no warm feelings.

Example 3

Another old man who also suffered from an incurable cancer had been admitted to hospital. He had not been told about the diagnosis, and before the ward round the nurse asked the doctor to do so. The doctor, who knew the patient well, asked 'Why?', and the nurse replied that it would be best for the patient to know the truth. The point was that the doctor had tried to tell the patient several times, but whenever she approached the topic of his disease he interrupted her and started to talk about something else. Therefore, the doctor had concluded that he did not want to be told. The nurse fully agreed that the doctor's interpretation of the patient's behaviour was correct, but she maintained that the patient should be told for his own sake.

This is an example of a modern phenomenon which aptly may be labelled neo-paternalism. According to the principle of autonomy this patient should not be told, because, as an autonomous person, he had the right to refuse information. The nurse was a paternalist, and perhaps she had also, as some people do, twisted the principle of autonomy to mean that people have some sort of duty to be informed and to act autonomously.

Example 4

The Samaritan principle, of course, refers to the parable of the Good Samaritan. A man had been attacked by robbers and left half-dead on the road; then the Samaritan came along, offered first-aid and paid for the man to be cared for at the local inn. This was a case of genuine paternalism as the word half-dead must mean that the robbed man was unconscious. However, it is tempting to write a modern version of the parable: the man wakes up when he sees the Samaritan and says: 'I do not want your help'. Then the Samaritan would have to make sure that the man was fully conscious and autonomous, and, if that was the case, he would, according to our ethical norms, have to take his donkey and ride on. In Denmark the health authorities admonish doctors that patients have the right to refuse treatment and the British Medical Association has done the same [173]. The deontological consideration takes priority over the consequential ones.

The following case resembles the revised parable. A young woman suffers a large haemorrhage during labour. She is a Jehovah's witness and she made it quite clear, already on admission, that she wanted no blood transfusions. She repeated this wish when she started to bleed. The doctors decided not to act against her wish, even when she became unconscious, and the woman died.

This tragic case is interesting from the point of view that it revealed the ambiguity of the ethical norms of the Danish society. A few days later, one of the leading national newspapers wrote in an editorial that the doctors at this hospital had committed murder. The ethical norms in our societies are changing and at a given time both old and new norms prevail. This is one reason why the medical profession, no matter how they act, cannot avoid being met with moral indignation by some members of the community.

Needless to say, the situation would have been entirely different if the bleeding patient had been a child. Then genuinely paternalistic action would have been required, even against the parents' wishes.

Example 5

An old woman who was physically weak, but not senile, had just had influenza and was severely dehydrated. She said several times that she was tired of life and wished to die. She did not want anything to drink, and she certainly did not want an intravenous drip. The doctor and the staff nurse in unison tried to persuade her that she would feel very much better if she was rehydrated, but she did not change her mind.

In the end the doctor and the nurse decided to overrule her clearly expressed wish. They simply said that it was necessary to put up a drip and did so in spite of her protestations and weak resistance. An observer would have had to conclude that this was a blatant violation of the principle of respect for autonomy, but, after having been rehydrated, the patient regained her zest for life and was very happy when she was discharged from hospital.

In retrospect, one may argue that this was a case of justified genuine paternalism in a temporarily non-autonomous patient, but when the doctor and the nurse made the decision they could not have been sure that the story would have such a happy ending. The patient might have died of old age after some days or weeks, and in that case one would have said that they prolonged her suffering by violating her autonomous wish.

Example 6

A young woman is admitted to hospital suffering from ulcerative colitis. She has had the disease for a long time and has received adequate treatment. Now, she is in a bad condition in spite of that treatment, and a course of corticosteroids has had no appreciable effect. It is concluded that it is necessary to do a total colectomy to save her life, but the patient refuses surgical treatment. She says that she does not wish to run the risk of having to have an ileostomy for life. She is told that, probably, it will be possible to restore the normal anatomy by a pouch operation, but that does not make her change her mind. The medical staff use all their powers of persuasion and remind her of her responsibilities towards her two children, but she still refuses. She remains fully conscious and fully aware of her situation. Then, after two weeks, she gives in, saying: 'You leave me no choice', and the colectomy is done. This story also had a happy ending. The patient recovered and fully accepted the treatment she had been given.

One may say that this case presented no serious ethical problem. The doctors gave the patient all the information she needed, and they respected her right to self-determination, as they did not, of course, do the colectomy until the patient had consented. However, we still have to ask to what extent the doctors respected her autonomy. An autonomous decision is a decision which is made without external coercion and in this case the doctors and nurses exposed the patient to maximal psychological pressure. However, most doctors will say, just as the patient did afterwards, that the medical staff acted correctly, and the example shows that good clinical practice often requires an element of paternalism [174].

Example 7

A middle-aged woman with a duodenal ulcer was seen as an out-patient by a gastroenterologist. At that time this disease could only be treated by lowering the gastric acid production by means of an H_2-receptor antagonist or a proton pump inhibitor, and the latter of these drugs was very expensive. It was known from randomized clinical trials that the cheapest H_2-blocker (cimetidine) healed about 75% of ulcers within four weeks, whereas the proton pump inhibitor healed almost all ulcers. The drug expenses were partly covered by the health service, and it was the policy of that department always to start treatment with cimetidine and to reserve the new drug for that minority of cases who did not respond. This patient did not accept this policy. She had heard about the new drug and demanded that it was prescribed to her from the start.

Consider, once again, the three questions from the first example. From a patient-orientated consequentialist point of view (question 1) there can be no doubt that it would be better, but only marginally so, to receive the new drug from the start. From the deontological point of view (question 3) one might argue that it is the patient's right to decide for herself, but the situation is not quite that simple. Respect for autonomy implies a right to be informed and a right to refuse treatment, but it does not necessarily imply a right to receive any treatment. A person with a common cold, for instance, cannot demand that her doctor writes a prescription for penicillin. But, of course, in this case the woman's wish carries some weight.

The important question is the second one. What would happen to the health service if all doctors started prescribing the expensive drug in such a case? It would obviously cost a lot of money and, since any public health service has a limited budget, it would mean that the money would have to be saved in some other way. The real cost is not one of pounds sterling or euros, but the *opportunity cost*, i.e. the lost opportunities somewhere else in the health service. Doctors employed by a national health service have a duty towards all patients seeking the help of the service, and they are co-responsible for the fair distribution of the limited resources.

The doctor balanced these considerations and decided to maintain that she would only write a prescription for the cheaper drug. She also felt that the patient's wish was somewhat immoral, as those patients who use the facilities of a public health service should also respect that the resources must be distributed as fairly as possible.

Example 8

Many of the inhabitants at a nursing home for old people suffered from senile dementia, and from time to time one of them left the home and wandered helplessly round the roads of the neighbourhood. Once, when an old woman had done so, the police were contacted, and the officer on duty was willing to send a patrol car round to look for her, but he stressed that they were only allowed to ask her whether she wanted to go home. They would have to respect her right to self-determination.

The nursing home was reasonably well staffed, but they could not prevent such incidents. They could not possibly watch the front door all the time, and in the end they decided to install a combination lock. Those who wished to leave the home would have to press a four-figure number, which would be easy to do for anybody who was not severely demented. That initiative, how-ever, caused a local political uproar. Some politicians said that the old peoples' autonomy had been violated.

Both the policeman's remark and the reaction of the politicians are good examples of absurd misinterpretations of the concepts of autonomy and the right to self-determination. Obviously, the senile inhabitants of the nursing home were not autonomous, and the installation of the combination lock was an act of genuine paternalism. It may be argued from a legal point of view that these people had not been declared incapable of managing their own affairs and that no guardians had been appointed, but, as mentioned above, one should distinguish between law and ethics.

It is peculiar that well-meant and usually quite justified paternalism within the health service causes so much debate when few people object to the com-pulsory use of safety straps or crash-helmets. Those regulations are good examples of unsolicited paternalism.

Example 9

A 60-year-old man with advanced lung cancer and bone metastases was treated with long-acting opiates orally, but pain relief was quite inadequate. Therefore, a moderate dose of morphine was added to the intravenous drip with some effect. Gradually, the dose was increased and after a few hours the patient was virtually pain-free. The dose was increased no further. Twelve hours later he died.

Most doctors would approve of the treatment of this patient. It could not be excluded, nor proved, that the treatment had shortened his life, but the aim of the treatment was to relieve his distress. The duty to preserve life weighs heavily among the deontological considerations, but as mentioned earlier no deontological principle is absolute, and on balance it seems right to have treated the patient in this way.

Then imagine that this patient some months earlier, when he began to feel the pain from the metastases and the diagnosis was first made, had asked his doctor to put an end to his life. He did not want to live through the last few months and his wife agreed with him. The doctor refused as she did not wish to commit a crime, but she also asked herself, 'Should euthanasia be legalized?'

Consider the first of our three standard questions. Would it be best for the patient to die at that time? To help us answer this question we may imagine that the patient on his way home from the doctor had a myocardial infarction and died. In that case both the doctor and the family would probably have said that it was a merciful end to his life, so probably the answer to that question is 'yes'. Then consider the third question. Should we not respect this wish of an autonomous person? As mentioned already (example 7), patients cannot demand any treatment from their doctor and that must include euthanasia, and a doctor cannot be expected to act contrary to her own moral norms. But one might argue that a doctor who approves of euthanasia should be allowed to comply with the patient's wish.

The second question, i.e. the question of the universal consequences, is the one which worries us most. Legalization would have the effect that all patients with incurable cancer, as well as their relatives, would suffer the additional burden of having to decide whether or not euthanasia was the right solution. Euthanasia is accepted in the Netherlands, and a Dutch woman, whose husband had cancer, once said that she had been given the choice between being her husband's murderer or his torturer!

The slippery slope argument must also be taken into account. The acceptance of euthanasia in incurable cancer might gradually lead to the acceptance of this practice in other categories of patients. There is already one Dutch example of euthanasia in the case of a divorced middle-aged woman who had lost both her children and could no longer see the purpose of her life [175]. Possibly, the practice might also be extended to old people who are in a poor state. Such patients sometimes express a wish to die and then explain that they do not wish this for their own sake, but because they are such a burden to their children.

These nine examples serve to illustrate the principles of ethical reasoning in clinical practice, but clinicians, of course, also face many other ethical dilemmas. Many of these are well analysed in the BMA publication *Medical Ethics Today* [27].

Clinical research ethics

Clinical research is a useful activity in society. People expect that medicine progresses, and that more and more diseases will be amenable to efficient treatment. There is a great need for both basic research and clinical research, including the critical assessment of new and existing diagnostic and therapeutic methods. Each type of research presents ethical problems of its own, but here we shall only consider some of the general principles.

In one respect research ethics differs fundamentally from the ethics of clinical practice. The medical practitioner may sometimes feel the tension between paternalism and respect for autonomy, but if she acts within the grey area between morally justified paternalism and unsolicited paternalism, there is no doubt that she does so to benefit her patient as much as possible. The doctor who violates her patient's right to information and self-determination does so for the patient's own sake.

Clinical researchers also wish to help sick people, but the people they benefit are not primarily those patients who are enrolled in the trials, but future patients. Therefore, the researcher who does not inform the participants of a trial adequately and secures their consent, does not act paternalistically; she just violates their autonomy in order to help somebody else. It is the patients themselves who must decide whether or not they wish to behave altruistically. In the past, doctors did not always ask for their patients' consent, but now it is required by the Helsinki Declaration of the World Medical Association [176] and in some countries by law, and it is also required that all research involving human subjects is approved by a research ethics committee. The structure of the committee system varies from country to country. In many countries it is considered sufficient that each institution establishes a committee of its own, whereas in Denmark a nation-wide independent system of regional committees has been established.

The patients are entitled to both written and verbal information, and it is one of the responsibilities of the ethics committees to ensure that the written information is adequate. Unfortunately, many researchers have great difficulties explaining in plain language without technical terms what their project is about and what it involves from the participants' point of view. The length of the information sheets also varies. In the United States they are very long and detailed as they include a lot of the background documentation, perhaps to protect doctors and drug companies rather than the patients, whereas they are shorter in Europe, but not necessarily less informative from the patients' point of view.

Research on unconscious, mentally ill or other non-autonomous patients present particular ethical problems, and sometimes consent by proxy is required, but here we shall confine ourselves to research on autonomous persons who can decide for themselves whether or not they wish to participate. When we ask such patients why they wish to take part, we usually get the answer that they do so to benefit future patients. They feel that they themselves benefit from previous research where other patients offered their assistance, and now they accept that it is their turn. This is a very important point as it follows that research which will not benefit future patients is ethically questionable. Research projects which are methodologically flawed are, of course, always unethical as unreliable results will not benefit anybody, and it ought to be one of the duties of ethics committees to ensure that such projects are never launched. However, there are also those projects which, in spite of the fact that they are methodologically acceptable, are not likely to benefit future patients. Drug firms, for instance, often wish to test new products, which are likely to be as good as, but not better than those marketed by their competitors. This is of course a legitimate enterprise from a commercial point of view, but one may argue that the doctor who asks his patients to participate is betraying their trust. The patients accept on the implicit assumption that they are helping other patients, but the only ones who are benefited are, in fact, the drug company and perhaps the doctor who may receive financial support from the company for future research.

Randomized trials are, of course, also unethical if the problem in question has already been adequately solved by previous trials, and as mentioned before (p. 142) the protocol for a randomized trial should always include a meta-analysis of previous studies. This procedure would also rule out those unnecessary trials which drug firms sometimes initiate in some country in order to disseminate knowledge of their product in that particular market.

Patients who take part in randomized trials do so on trust. They trust that their doctor will take care of them during the trials and they also trust that the project is worthwhile. Therefore, it is the duty of the doctor who asked them to participate to ensure that the trial is acceptable from a methodological point of view, and she cannot delegate that responsibility to a drug firm. One cannot, of course, expect that all doctors, taking part in a multicentre trial, will possess sufficient knowledge about sample size calculations, statistical tests, the handling of drop-outs, etc. to be able to judge for themselves all aspects of the quality of the trial, but then they must make sure that the drug firm has handed over the full responsibility for the trial to an independent, sufficiently qualified steering committee. This committee should be in possession of all the scientific data, and it is their responsibility that the results are published as soon as possible after the conclusion of the trial. The drug firm must not be able to postpone or prevent publication if the trial did not give the desired result.

This does not mean that the doctors responsible for the trial should ignore the expertise of the drug firms. Many firms employ highly qualified methodologists and statisticians, and they should of course be consulted at all stages of the project. It must also be appreciated that a drug firm has a responsibility of its own, as regards the quality of the project. It is well known that doctors running a trial do not always do so with sufficient discipline, and there are sad examples of fraud where doctors have 'invented' patients. Therefore, it is both the right and the duty of the company to monitor the running of the trial at all centres at regular intervals.

Admittedly, many of those trials which are done today do not fulfil these requirements, but they would, if doctors had made it a precondition for their participation.

The majority of clinicians are not actively engaged in research, but they may get involved if they see a patient who takes part in a trial. The patient may have been admitted to hospital as an emergency because of a different disease, or she may have decided to consult her general practitioner for some reason or other. In all such cases the doctor who sees the patient must immediately contact the colleagues running the trial in order to ensure that nothing is done inadvertently which interferes with the protocol. Most clinical researchers have experienced the situation when a patient was lost to their trial because some colleague did not bother to contact them and just told the patient that she had better stop taking the trial medicine for the time being.

CHAPTER 8

Critical Reading of Medical Journals

Can clinicians and statisticians be friends?
[Buchanan & Smythe [177]]

Rational diagnosis and treatment must be based on the results of clinical research, and readers of medical journals must know enough about research methods and statistics to assess critically the papers that appear in the medical journals. This chapter is a brief guide to help critical readers not to be misled by methodological flaws, hidden sources of bias and misleading statistical calculations [14,178,179]. Those who wish to know more about these topics must consult textbooks on research methods, clinical epidemiology and biostatistics [1–17].

Logical analysis of medical papers

The best advice which we can offer the critical reader of a medical paper is to start by analysing its logical structure. Most research projects aim at establishing causal relationships, and it is possible to distinguish between three different approaches:

1 The scientist reasons forward in time, from cause to effect. The project aims at establishing a connection between a particular phenomenon (the cause) and future phenomena (the effects). The results of the study are conditional probabilities of the type P(effect|cause). Prospective cohort studies are typical examples of this type of reasoning.

2 The scientist reasons backward in time, from effect to cause. The project aims at establishing a connection between a particular phenomenon (the effect) and past phenomena (the causes). The results of the study are conditional probabilities of the type P(cause|effect). Retrospective case–control studies are typical examples.

3 The scientist analyses to what extent different phenomena are associated with one another, but is unable to determine the direction of causality. He cannot be sure what causes what. This problem typically arises in cross-sectional studies, i.e. studies where all observations are made at the same time.

The *prospective cohort study* represents the first of the three types of scientific logic. One or more groups of persons who fulfil a well-defined set of criteria are selected and are then observed for a period of time. These groups of people are also called cohorts (from Latin *cohors*, originally a Roman army unit consisting of 300–600 legionaries), and they are studied prospectively in the sense that all the observations take place during the study according to a detailed protocol.

Some prognostic studies only comprise one cohort. One may, for instance, select a cohort of patients with hypertension (the cause) and then record the incidence of cerebrovascular attacks (the effect) during the study period. This design, however, permits no comparisons and it would be much more informative to compare the observations in this cohort with those in a comparable cohort of normotensive persons.

The randomized clinical trial is a special type of prospective cohort study where, in contrast to simple prognostic studies, the causal factor is introduced by active intervention and the patients are allocated at random to two cohorts. This type of research which represents the gold standard for testing new treatments was discussed in detail in Chapter 6.

The *retrospective case–control study* also serves to analyse causal relationships, but the procedure is very different. Two groups of persons are selected: the cases and the controls. The cases are characterized by presenting the effect in question, typically a particular disease, and the controls are characterized by the absence of this effect, typically normal subjects. The frequency of the assumed causal factor is recorded in both groups and the reasoning is backwards in time from effect to cause. A paediatrician who wishes to investigate the relationship between splenectomy after abdominal trauma and the later development of pneumococcal sepsis might record the frequency of a history of splenectomy in a sample of children with pneumococcal sepsis (the cases) and then compare this frequency with that in a comparable group of children without pneumococcal sepsis (the controls). The detection of a difference between these frequencies would suggest a causal relationship, but it would not tell him anything about the magnitude of the risk of developing a sepsis after splenectomy. This type of case–control study is labelled retrospective as it incorporates information (the history of splenectomy) that was recorded before the start of the study.

The difference between cohort studies and case–control studies is

Table 13 Cohort and case–control studies. If the data represent the results of a comparative cohort study, the table is read horizontally. a/(a+b) and c/(c+d) are calculated, i.e. the probability that members of the two cohorts develop the effect. If the data represent the results of a case–control study, the table is read vertically. a/(a+c) and b/(b+d) are calculated, i.e. the probability that cases and controls presented the alleged causal factor.

		Effect +	Effect −	Total
	+	a	b	a + b
Cause	−	c	d	c + d
	Total	a + c	b + d	1000

illustrated by Table 13, which shows that the two designs require different calculations. The results of cohort studies are often analysed by determining the relative risk, RR, which is the ratio between P(effect|cause) in the two groups (cf. p. 136). It is calculated as follows:

$$RR = \frac{a/(a+b)}{c/(c+d)}$$

Case-control studies do not permit such 'horizontal' calculations in the fourfold table as the number of cases and the number of controls were decided upon by the researcher. Instead the odds ratio (OR) is calculated, according to this formula:

$$OR = \frac{a/c}{b/d} = \frac{ad}{bc}$$

The OR serves as a good approximation to the relative risk if the frequency of the effect is very small, i.e. $a << (a + b)$ and $c << (c + d)$.

These two types of studies present both advantages and disadvantages. Prospective cohort studies are by far the most reliable, as all observations take place during the study according to a fixed protocol, but they are laborious and expensive if the cohorts are large and the observation period long. They permit the demonstration of several effects of one cause, and the interpretation of the results is usually quite simple. However, the vaccination project which was discussed on p. 58 illustrates that sometimes it may be difficult to distinguish between real causes, common causes and concomitant causal factors. Confounding problems of that kind are only excluded in unbiased randomized trials.

Retrospective case–control studies are much easier to do, and sometimes they represent the only option. It would, for example, be impossible to establish an association between rare congenital malformations and the ingestion of certain drugs during pregnancy in any other way. Case–control studies may be used to demonstrate several causes of one effect, but it is always difficult to reconstruct what happened in the past, and retrospective research is much more sensitive to confounding than prospective studies. Case–control studies present many other problems, some of which deserve special mention.

Problems of case–control research

Case–control studies, just like other scientific studies, require meticulous planning. It is necessary to write a protocol which states the hypotheses to be tested, the necessary definitions, and the in- and exclusion criteria for choosing the cases and the controls. Sometimes, however, no such detailed protocol is prepared [180] and for that reason alone the results of the study may be difficult to interpret.

It is particularly important to choose a relevant control group and to ensure that the cases and the controls are sufficiently comparable, but that is not always easy. In studies aimed at determining the causes of a particular disease it may be useful to compare patients with the disease with patients suspected of the disease. For instance, women with breast cancer diagnosed by mammography may be compared with women who were referred to mammography on the suspicion of cancer, but did not have the disease. However, even this procedure is not safe. Malignant and benign breast lesions may have some causal factors in common and the study may produce false negative results.

The reliability of data that have been collected retrospectively is often doubtful. The note in an old hospital record that some patient was subjected to a splenectomy is undoubtedly true, but the information that a patient suffered from pneumonia, rheumatoid arthritis or diarrhoea, or that he presented a duodenal ulcer at endoscopy, is much less reliable, as the diagnostic criteria used in the daily routine are rarely very precise. In most cases registers of diagnoses and causes of death are also unreliable [181] and they should not be used for research purposes unless they have been validated.

Information about past events is particularly unreliable when it depends on the memory of the participants in the study. If, for instance, a group of patients with ulcerative colitis and a group of healthy persons are asked whether or not they have ever suffered from eczema, it is only to be expected that the patients, who are more interested in the possible causes of the disease than the controls, will search their memory more thoroughly. Such *recall bias* may easily lead to a difference between the recorded rates of eczema in the two groups.

The interview technique may also be a source of bias. If, for example, the group of cases is interviewed before the group of controls, the interviews of the controls may be less thorough than those of the cases, because the interviewer grew tired, or they may be more thorough, because the interviewer gradually improved his technique. Preferably, cases and controls should be interviewed in random order, but that is rarely done.

'Blinding' is also a realistic option in many case–control studies. The interviewer need not know which of the interviewed persons are cases and which are controls, and, by including irrelevant questions in the questionnaires, both interviewers and patients may be kept ignorant of the hypotheses to be tested.

The medical literature illustrates only too well the importance of these and many other methodological problems, as there is no limit to causal associations which have been 'proved' by case–control studies. A series of studies, for instance, suggested a connection between a history of induced abortion and the development of breast cancer, and a much quoted meta-analysis concluded that the risk increase was 30% (corresponding to an odds ratio of 1.3 with 95% confidence interval 1.2–1.4) [182]. A Swedish team, however, found no association (odds ratio 0.95) and, when they consulted a register recording all abortions and corrected the information provided by the women, they even found that abortion had a protective effect, the risk of cancer being reduced by 37% (odds ratio 0.63) [183]. Recently, a large Danish cohort study, including 1.5 million women, conclusively exploded these myths, as it was found that the relative risk was 1.00 (95% confidence interval 0.94–1.06) [184]. It remains to explain these differences, but probably recall bias played an important role in the first study, as the women with breast cancer may have been more willing than the controls to admit that they had had an abortion. In this way case–control studies often give rise to false alarms, and it has been recommended that one should not pay too much attention to studies which suggest the harmful effect of some factor, if the risk increase is less than 100% (i.e. the odds ratio is less than 2). It follows that the case–control design cannot be used to test new treatments, as in most cases the expected effect is much smaller than the likely sources of bias.

Other designs

Cross-sectional studies are the easiest ones to do. Data from one or more groups of people are collected at one moment in time, and the association between them is analysed by means of appropriate statistical tests. It may, however, be difficult to establish what is the cause and what is the effect, as illustrated by the difficulties of determining the relationship between *Helicobacter pylori* infection and the development of duodenal ulcers, or that between unemployment and alcoholism (p. 59). In other cases, only one interpretation is possible. If, for example, an association is found between a certain tissue type and the occurrence of rheumatoid arthritis, it is, of course, the tissue type which predisposes to arthritis and not the arthritis which changes the tissue type.

One should also watch out for longitudinal interpretations of cross-sectional data. Once a textbook provided the information that the prevalence of intermittent claudication was 1.4% in 40–49-year-old men and 7.0% in 70–79 year olds. In women, the corresponding figures were 1.9% and 1.0%. A longitudinal interpretation of these data, taken at face value, would mean that throughout life more and more men developed the disease, whereas more and more women were cured. It was, however, not a cohort study where the same people had been observed for 30 years, but two sets of cross-sectional data from different populations, and the high incidence among younger women probably reflects that during the last few decades more young women have adopted the habit of smoking.

It has also been shown in cross-sectional studies that the frequency of *Helicobacter* infection of the stomach is correlated to age (in such a way that approximately 30% of 30-year-old men and 60% of 60-year olds are infected and so forth), and a longitudinal interpretation would suggest that throughout their lives more and more people get infected. Most people, however, are infected when they are quite young, and the association between the prevalence and the age reflects that for many years the risk of infection has decreased.

Cross-sectional studies are also associated with other sources of error. Once it was found that gall stones were diagnosed more frequently in duodenal ulcer patients than in patients without abdominal complaints. Did that mean that gall stones predisposed to duodenal ulcers or that duodenal ulcers predisposed to gall stones? Probably neither of these explanations were true. The ulcer patients who sought medical advice because of their abdominal pain were frequently examined for gall stones before the ulcer diagnosis was made, and sometimes the investigation led to the demonstration of stones which caused no symptoms at all.

Similarly, it was once reported in a study of hospital patients that the rate of previous admissions to psychiatric institutions was higher among ulcer patients than in the background population, and it was suggested that psychological factors played a causal role in the development of this disease. However, it is also possible that duodenal ulcer patients with a psychiatric history were more liable to reach the hospital threshold (p. 61) than duo-denal ulcer patients with no psychiatric problems. Such misinterpretation of cross-sectional data is known as *Berkson's fallacy* [185], which commonly appears in medical journals.

This presentation of different designs is by no means exhaustive. Hybrids exist, especially the retrospective or historical cohort study. A surgeon, for instance, may wish to study his successes and failures with a particular surgical operation. He goes through the hospital notes at his unit from the past few years and, assuming that the patients were seen routinely in the out-patient department for a period of time, he records the results of the operation. This is a retrospective study in the sense that the data collection took place before the start of the study, but it is also a cohort study as the surgeon reasoned from cause (surgical operation) to effect (result of operation). This design shares the strength of other cohort studies that it permits the calculation of P(effect|cause), but it also shares the weakness of other retrospective studies that the data quality may be poor. The indications for doing the operation were not defined in advance and stated in a detailed protocol, and probably the notes in the patients' records about the clinical status after the operation were quite unstructured. Therefore, the scientific value of such studies is limited, but the results may be of some use for the purpose of ordinary quality control.

A different hybrid is seen when case–control studies are done within the framework of a large randomized trial in order to explore the causes of rare adverse effects. Such studies are prospective in the sense that they use data that have been collected in connection with the randomized trial, but the logic is that of other case–control studies, i.e. reasoning from effect to cause.

Finally, it may be noted that the terms prospective and retrospective are somewhat ambiguous. In this presentation they refer to the time of the data collection. Others identify prospective research with reasoning from cause to effect (i.e. cohort logic) and retrospective research with reasoning from effect to cause (i.e. case–control logic). This ambiguity is unfortunate as it is necessary to distinguish between those strengths and weaknesses that reflect the time of the data collection and those that reflect the logical structure of the research project.

Descriptive statistics

The attitude of doctors towards statistics ranges from distrust to blind faith. Some dismiss statistical calculations as superfluous, arguing that a signal which is not sufficiently strong to be recognized without statistical hocus-pocus must be uninteresting, whereas others accept any result as long as it is supported by a *P*-value below 5%. This spectrum of attitudes probably reflects that the teaching of statistics in many medical schools is either too limited or too theoretical. Some years ago a survey among Danish doctors revealed that the majority did not know the correct interpretation of such basic concepts as a *P*-value, a standard deviation (SD) and a standard error (SE) [29], and probably the situation is much the same elsewhere.

The simplest form of statistics is concerned with the description and presentation of the data. The researcher cannot publish all his observations but must process and condense the results in such a way that as little information as possible is lost. He may, for instance, have studied a sample of 19 patients with hyperthyroidism and instead of publishing all the crude data shown in Table 14, he will make brief statements of the following kind:

Ophthalmopathy was found in 37% of the patients. This trivial statement shows that data processing always entails some loss of information. If the statement is read out of context, we cannot know if the experience is based on only 19 or on many more patients. The example also shows that the method of data

Table 14 Data from 19 patients with hyperthyroidism. The patients have been listed according to their serum thyroxin concentration.

Age (years)	Ophthalmopathy (+ or −)	Severity of symptoms (Dr NN's clinical index)	Serum thyroxin (nmol/L)			
59	−	8	126			
35	−	23	127			
51	+	14	131			
62	−	7	137			
43	−	23	146	←	Lower quartile	⌐
62	+	8	155			
32	−	20	157			
40	−	16	167			
44	+	10	171			Inter-
58	−	28	175	←	Median	quartile
54	+	9	179			range
38	−	27	185			
76	−	14	218			
36	−	22	243			
55	−	34	250	←	Upper quartile	⌐
43	+	25	256			
50	+	33	269			
22	−	35	333			
27	+	29	397			

processing depends on the level of measurement of the original data. The presence or absence of ophthalmopathy constitutes a binary scale (p. 11), and a series of observations on that level are conventionally condensed to a rate in per cent.

The mean age of the patients was 46.7 years (SD 13.7). The age of a patient is recorded on an interval scale (p. 11), and the researcher condensed the 19 observations by calculating the mean and the standard deviation (SD).

The calculation and interpretation of the standard deviation was explained on p. 23, and Fig. 3 illustrated that the interval, delimited by the mean ± 2 standard deviations, encompasses 95% of the observations provided that the distribution is Gaussian. Therefore, if this requirement is fulfilled, the reader may expect that the age of almost all patients in this small sample ranged from about 19 to about 74 years. Table 14 shows that this is not far from the truth as the youngest patient was 22 and the oldest 76 years. In other words the standard deviation serves to visualize the distribution of the original data. There is, however, one problem: biological distributions are rarely Gaussian and the reader who interprets the standard deviation in this way may be seriously misled.

Therefore, it would be no loss if editors of medical journals banned the use of the standard deviation altogether and instead recommended the next method to be explained.

The median concentration of serum thyroxine was 175 nmol/L, the total range was 126–397 nmol/L, and the interquartile range was 146–250 nmol/L. The concentration of thyroxine was also recorded on an interval scale, but the author chose not to calculate the mean and standard deviation. Instead he ranked the data, as shown in Table 14, and determined the quartiles by dividing the sample into four equal parts. The three quartiles are called the lower quartile, the median (or half-way value) and the upper quartile, and the range between the lower to the upper quartile is denoted the interquartile range.

The quartiles are special cases of *quantiles*. If the ranked results are divided up into 10 groups, the nine values at which the divisions occur are called deciles, and if a sufficiently large number of results are divided up into 100 groups the divisions are called percentiles. Sometimes other quantiles are used. When discussing the calculation of the normal range (p. 31) it was suggested that the highest and the lowest fortieth (or 2.5%) of the results were removed, the remaining observations constituting the *observed 95% range*. The interquartile range (for small samples) and the observed 95% range (for large samples) are better measures of the dispersion of the results than the total range, which may be influenced by a single, atypically extreme value. It is often necessary to perform interpolations when quantiles are determined;

thus the median of 10 results (in ranking order) must be calculated as the average of the 5th and the 6th result.

The measurements of the serum thyroxine concentrations constitute an interval scale and therefore the author might have quoted the mean rather than the median concentration, but it would have been quite misleading to quote the standard deviation, as the distribution is not Gaussian; it is positively skew and resembles the distribution shown in Fig. 5(a). Calculation of mean ± 2 standard deviations gives the result 201 ± 148 nmol/L, suggesting that almost all observations lay within the interval 53–349 nmol/L, which, as seen in Table 14, was not the case.

Doctor NN's clinical index was used to measure the severity of the patients' symptoms. The median score was 22, the total range 7–35, and the interquartile range 10–28. This statement is analogous to the previous one, and if the reader ranks the scores in Table 14, he will find that the statement is correct. A clinical index constitutes an ordinal scale (p. 11), as it must be taken for granted that the symptoms of a patient with a high score are more severe than those of a patient with a lower score, but it cannot be assumed that the relationship is linear and that the index also constitutes an interval scale. Therefore, it would have made little sense to calculate the mean, which requires an interval scale, and the standard deviation, which requires both an interval scale and a Gaussian distribution. This mistake is often found in medical papers.

In summary, these examples illustrate that the researcher condenses the original observations by the calculation of so-called statistics, and the choice of statistic depends on the level of measurement of the data. The minimum requirements are the following:

Statistic	Level of measurement
Rate	Nominal scale
Median and quantiles	Ordinal scale
Mean	Interval scale
Standard deviation	Interval scale and Gaussian distribution

It is, of course, always possible to reduce the level of measurement. In one of the examples the researcher reduced the interval measurements of thyroxine in nmol/L to an ordinal scale by ranking, determining the median and the quartiles, and he could have reduced the level of measurement even further to a binary (nominal) scale by distinguishing only between 'high' and 'low' concentrations. It is not permissible, however, to increase the level of measurement, which he would have done if he had calculated the mean and the standard deviation of the clinical index.

Estimation

The rate of ophthalmopathy was 37% (95% confidence interval: 16% to 62%). Figure 14 shows that seven of the 19 patients suffered from ophthalmopathy, which means that the observed rate was 37%. The clinician, however, also wanted to estimate the 'true' rate, and for that purpose he calculated the 95% confidence interval. In statistical terminology the observed rate, which refers to the sample in question, is an example of a statistic, whereas the unknown 'true' rate, which refers to the underlying population, is an example of a *population parameter*. Therefore, the calculation of a confidence interval is also called interval estimation of a parameter. We introduce this terminology as the use of such expressions is one of the major stumbling blocks when doctors wish to study textbooks on biostatistics.

The principle of estimation or calculation of confidence intervals was explained on pp. 102–6, and here we shall only recapitulate briefly that in the long run we may expect to be right 19 out of 20 times when we conclude that the population parameter (the 'true' rate) lies within the calculated interval. It was also emphasized, however, that this does not necessarily mean that we may be 95% confident that the true value lies within the interval in the individual case. We must take into account all available evidence about the problem in question. Perhaps the rate of ophthalmopathy was much lower in other studies of similar patients, and perhaps our study was one of the rare cases where the confidence interval did not catch the true value.

The mean age of the 19 patients was 46.7 years (SE 3.1). This statement resembles the descriptive statement, mean ± 2 standard deviations discussed above, but the meaning is very different. SE or SEM is the standard error of the mean, and it is calculated by means of this very simple formula where N is the number of patients:

$$SE = SD/\sqrt{N}$$

The standard error is of some interest to readers of medical papers as it permits them to calculate the confidence interval for the mean. For practical purposes the 95% confidence interval of the 'true' mean is the sample mean ± 2 SE, and in this case this interval is 40.5–52.9 years.

In many cases the SE is quoted when the reader is not the least interested in knowing the confidence interval, but wishes to assess the dispersion of the results. It is the standard deviation, not the standard error, which serves that purpose, but of course it is quite easy to calculate 2 SD, if SE is known, using the reverse formula: 2 SD = 2 SE × √N. It follows, as mentioned above, that the interval mean ± 2 SD is 19–75 years.

The mean thyroxine concentration was 201 nmol/L (SE 17). This statement is analogous to the previous one, but in spite of that it is misleading. The standard error cannot be used to calculate the confidence interval if the sample is small and if the distribution is markedly non-Gaussian. In this case the sample only comprised 19 patients and the distribution was skew to the right and, consequently, the reader cannot be very confident that the true mean lies within the interval 201 nmol/L ± 34 nmol/L. It can, however, be shown that the Gaussian assumption is less important if the sample is large, and the calculation might have been considered sufficiently reliable if the sample size had been, say, 100 patients. In our example it would have been better to calculate the median and the confidence interval of the median [186].

The resting pressure of the lower oesophageal sphincter in 25 healthy persons was 19 ± 3.0 mmHg (mean ± SE). Statements like this one are quite frequent in medical journals and the critical reader ought to realize at once that they are meaningless. The author only reported the value of 1 SE and it is easy to calculate that mean ± 2 SD = 19 ± 30 mmHg, which suggests that some of these subjects had a negative resting pressure. Obviously, the distribution was truncated and skew to the right as shown in Fig. 5(e), p. 31. Therefore, SD cannot be used to describe the distribution of the observations, and, as the sample was small, SE cannot be used to calculate the confidence interval.

Expressions of the type *mean ± a* are very common, and sometimes the author even forgets to tell the reader what *a* means, i.e. whether it is 1 SE, 2 SE, 1 SD or 2 SD. The same problem occurs in histograms and graphs where the 'uncertainty' of the results is indicated by a vertical line, but where the author forgets to tell the reader what the line means.

Confidence intervals may be calculated for many other statistics, e.g. the difference between two rates (p. 135), the difference between two means, relative risks and odds ratios [187].

Testing hypotheses

Both cohort studies and case-control studies are examples of hypothetico-deductive research. The scientist:

1 evolves a hypothesis as regards a possible cause–effect relationship;
2 plans and carries out a suitable trial or survey; and

3 tests to what extent the results of this trial or survey are compatible with the initial hypothesis.

Some researchers, however, do not adhere to this plan.

Pseudohypothetico-deductive logic

Imagine a person who is looking out of the window at a large car park that is divided up into two parking areas, one of which is better sheltered than the other. He notices the make, the size and the colour of the different cars, and suddenly he discovers that there are many more red cars in the sheltered area (11 out of 50) than in the other (two out of 48). He then does the appropriate statistical test (Fisher's exact test), finds that $P = 0.02$ and concludes, rather hastily, that owners of red cars prefer to park in a sheltered place. This is obviously a case of muddled thinking, but it is necessary to be able to pinpoint the flaw in the argument. The 'scientist' reversed the order of the first two steps of the sequence mentioned above. Presumably, he had no hypothesis in mind when he started to look at the cars. He more or less consciously noticed the distribution of Fords, Talbots, Volvos, blue cars, black cars, etc., and he only decided to do a significance test when he saw that the red cars were unevenly distributed. We are, both in our daily lives and in our research, witnesses to innumerable chance events, 5% of which are 'statistically significant' at the 5% level, 1% at the 1% level and so forth, and those who disregard this simple fact are prone to make hasty conclusions. The surprising fact is that many researchers indulge in this kind of *pseudohypothetico-deductive logic*. They make numerous observations and whenever they see something unusual they do a significance test and conclude that they have discovered a new regularity in nature.

We were referring to this kind of logic when we warned against 'fishing expeditions' on p. 137, but it also appears in other disguises. In recent years different types of multiple regression analyses have become very popular, but sometimes the results are interpreted rather uncritically. Perhaps numerous data are recorded when patients enter a prognostic cohort study, and then it is tempting to analyse afterwards, by means of a regression analysis, which of these characteristics were significantly correlated to the patients' prognosis. That, however, amounts to no more than a sophisticated 'fishing expedition', if it was not clearly stated in the protocol which hypotheses were to be tested.

The results of multiple significance testing should of course not be totally ignored, but their main purpose is the provision of ideas for future studies. There is only one exception to this rule. If the number of patients is very large, the sample may be divided into two, permitting the researcher to go fishing in one subsample, and testing the new ideas in the other. The association between a particular characteristic and the prognosis is likely to be true if it is statistically significant in both subsamples.

Wrong sampling unit

Clinical research is done on groups (samples) of patients and the sampling unit in the statistical analysis is one patient. In Table 6 (p. 67), for instance, it is assumed that there were 111 patients. If we had discovered, when reading the original paper more carefully, that in fact it only comprised 70 patients, 41 of whom had been examined twice, the calculation of diagnostic rates would have made no sense. In that case the sample unit would not have been one patient, but one ultrasound examination, and the observations would no longer have been mutually independent; one would have expected the second examination in most of the 41 cases to have given the same result as the first examination.

The same holds true of randomized trials. In the example illustrated by Table 10a (p. 130) it was taken for granted that we were dealing with 600 different patients. If the treatment was not curative and if some patients had entered the trial twice, the statistical calculations would also have made no sense. One would have expected that most of those patients who tried the treatment twice would have responded the same way both times.

These examples may sound rather trivial, but nevertheless this fallacy, which is called the *wrong sampling unit*, often appears in medical papers in different disguises. One may, for instance, encounter the vascular surgeon who examined 150 patients, of whom 80 had unilateral and 70 bilateral arterial insufficiency. He thought that the 'sample' consisted of 220 diseased legs and based his statistical calculations on that figure. That is of course wrong as two legs from the same person are not mutually independent. If one leg is under the influence of the patient's diabetes, so is the other. Probably the most extreme example is the randomized trial of 58 patients, where the unit used for the statistical analysis was not a patient, but a joint. Altogether 3944 joints had been examined, and the resulting P-value was 0.00000001 (or as it was stated in the paper: 0.979126×10^{-8}). Obviously, the units were not mutually independent: if in some patient the treatment had an effect on one tender joint, it probably also had an effect on the others.

Epidemiologists make similar mistakes. In population surveys the effect of preventive measures is often related to the number of treatment years, i.e. the sum of the number of years each person was treated. This method was once used in a study of malaria prophylaxis in Tanzania [188], and it was over-looked that the risk of infection of a diplomat living in Dar es Salaam for one year is not the same as that of 26 tourists spending a fortnight in a rural area under primitive conditions. The same criticism may be raised against studies of the effect of contraceptive measures, where the measure of effect is number of pregnancies per year.

Finally, we should mention cross-over trials (p. 124), where, for example, 50 patients receive two treatments in succession. Here it is not permissible to compare the 50 observations during treatment *A* with the 50 observations during treatment *B*, as these 100 observations are not mutually independent, but paired two by two. One must use special statistical tests (tests for paired observations) suited for this design, as mentioned below.

Sample size calculations

Authors of medical papers must state in the 'Methods' section how they did the calculation of the sample size. These calculations require that the researchers, at the planning stage, make up their minds about the hypothesis to be tested and the statistical specifications of the trial. Readers of medical journals need not, of course, be able to do such calculations themselves, but they should know the general principles, so that they can check that the trial fulfils the requirements of proper hypothetico-deductive research.

Assuming a binary measure of effect (e.g. cured/not cured), the researchers should consider at the planning stage the following three questions, the answers to which constitute the specifications of the trial:

1 What risk of committing a type I error (p. 131) are we willing to accept? This is the risk of concluding that the treatment effects differ when in fact they are identical, and the conventional answer is 5%. If, however, the new treatment is expensive and the disease not very serious, it might be more reasonable only to accept a type I error risk (significance level) of 1%, in order to minimize the risk of introducing the treatment if it is no better than the old one.

2 What therapeutic gain are we looking for? Obviously, the sample size would have to be very large if the researcher was looking for a difference between treatment effects of 1%, whereas only a small trial would be needed to detect a therapeutic gain of 40% or more. Once again, the answer depends on the clinical problem. If it is a question of life or death, it is important not to overlook small therapeutic gains, and in that case a large trial is needed.

3 What risk of committing a type II error are we willing to accept. We

may have decided when we answered question 2 that we were looking for a therapeutic gain of, say, 10%, but we must realize that there is always the risk that we end up with a statistically non-significant result even when the difference between the treatment results is 10% or more. How large may that risk be? Many researchers accept type II error risks of 20% or more, which is surprising. If the disease is serious, one may well argue that the type II error risk ought to be smaller than the type I error risk, and in most cases they ought to be of the same order of magnitude.

If these questions have been answered, and if it is possible to predict roughly the effect rate in the control group, it is easy calculate the necessary number of patients, using the proper statistical formula [16], a graph or a computer program.

Example: '*The trial was designed to have 80% power (with 2α = 0.05) to detect a difference between the cure rates of at least 10%, and the required sample size was 750 patients.*' This is a typical quote from the methods section of a report of a randomized trial. The answer to the first question, i.e. the significance level (which is often called 2α), was 5%, the answer to the second question was 10%, and the answer to the third question was 20% (the 'power' being 100% – type II error risk). The sample size calculation, using these specifications, showed that 750 patients were needed.

Dr N and Dr R

The sample size calculation, as described above, was done according to conventional statistical theory, but the reader of a medical paper who has to interpret the resulting P-values must adopt a wider perspective. This topic was discussed on pp. 132–4, where it was pointed out that the reader's confidence in a P-value also depends on his confidence in the null hypothesis. We shall now illustrate this important point by means of a fictitious example [189].

Imagine two clinical researchers, Dr N and Dr R. The former, Dr N, aspired to the *Nobel* prize, for which reason he evolved highly original (even far-fetched) hypotheses which he then tested by suitable trials. The latter, Dr R, only *repeated* the research of others. He developed no original ideas, but whenever he read about a trial in an international journal that had given a significant result, he wanted to see if he could reproduce that finding.

First, we shall look at Dr N's career as a researcher, and we shall assume (rather unrealistically) that he has done 1000 randomized clinical trials comparing two treatments. Further, we shall imagine that this series comprised 900 trials where the treatments were equal and 100 where one treatment was markedly better than the other. In real life, of course, we never know the truth, but the assumption fits Dr N's research strategy. He develops original ideas, and usually (9 out of 10 times) the idea is wrong.

We also make the assumption that Dr N accepts the conventional significance level of 5% and that his samples of patients were always so large that the chance of overlooking a true difference was only 10%. In other words, this series of trials was characterized by a type I error risk of 5% and a type II error risk of 10%. These assumptions permit us to construct the fourfold table shown in Table 15.

H_0 (the null hypothesis) was true in 900 trials, but we must expect that Dr N obtained a statistically significant result ($P \leq 0.05$), simply by chance, in 5% of these trials (i.e. in 45). H_A (the alternative hypothesis) was true in 100 trials, but, considering the type II error risk, we must expect that Dr N obtained a statistically non-significant result ($P > 0.05$) in 10% of these trials (i.e. in 10).

It then follows, as shown in Table 15, that Dr N obtained a statistically significant result in 135 trials, and that in 33% or 45 of these the null hypothesis was true. In other words, we can only be 67% confident that there is a difference between the treatments when Dr N finds a statistically significant difference. We can, however, rely on his non-significant results as the null hypothesis was true in 855/865 = 99% of those cases where he found that $P > 0.05$.

We may analyse Dr R's research career in exactly the same way. He had also done 1000 trials, but he had confined himself to repeating the research of others, and therefore it is reasonable to assume that most of those treatments which he compared had, in fact, different effects. For the sake of the numerical example, we shall say that the null hypothesis was true in only 100 trials and that the alternative hypothesis was true in 900 trials.

Assuming, as in the case of Dr N, that the type I error risk is 5% and the

Table 15 Dr N's research career.

		Truth		
		H_A	H_0	*Total*
Result of significance test	$P \leq 0.05$	90	45	*135*
	$P > 0.05$	10	855	*865*
	Total	*100*	*900*	*1000*

Table 16 Dr R's research career.

		Truth		
		H_A	H_0	*Total*
Result of	P ≤ 0.05	810	5	*815*
significance test	P > 0.05	90	95	*185*
	Total	*900*	*100*	*1000*

type II error risk 10%, we can illustrate Dr R's career by means of Table 16. In 5% of the 100 trials where H_0 was true he obtained a statistically significant result, and in 10% of the 900 trials where H_A was true he obtained a non-significant result.

It follows, as shown in the table, that Dr R obtained a statistically significant result in 815 trials and that in 5 (i.e. in less than 1%) of these trials the null hypothesis was true. Therefore, the results of Dr R must be interpreted very differently from those of Dr N as we can be more than 99% confident that there is a difference between the treatments when Dr R finds a statistically significant difference. Dr R's non-significant results, however, are not very informative as in those cases there is almost a 50% chance that the alternative hypothesis is true.

In other words, the records of Dr N and Dr R are similar from the perspective of conventional statistical theory as for both series of trials the type I error risk was 5% and the type II error risk 10%. Nevertheless, the records are very different from the point of view of the reader of their papers who wishes to make up his mind to what extent he can rely on their significant results.

These examples provide important clues to the interpretation of *P*-values from the reader's point of view. Whenever we read the report of, for instance, a randomized clinical trial, we must consider whether the study belongs to Dr N's or Dr R's universe (or to an even more extreme universe). If our prior confidence in the null hypothesis is high, due to theoretical considerations or the results of others, we may decide that the study belongs to Dr N's universe and we shall not believe too much in a statistically significant *P*-value. If, on the other hand, we have good reasons to believe that the two treatments have different effects, we may refer the study to Dr R's universe, and decide that, probably, the treatment is effective even when the *P*-value is, for example, 0.10.

This approach can also be used to illustrate the importance of the sample size. Usually, it is taken for granted that the interpretation of the P-value has nothing to do with the size of the study, but it is easy to show that, other things being equal, one should have less confidence in a significant P-value if the study is small. The smaller the size of the sample, the greater the risk of committing a type II error, and if the two treatment groups are very small (e.g. 20 patients in each), the risk of obtaining a non-significant P-value may be up to 75% even when one treatment is considerably better than the other. Table 17 shows what would have happened if Dr N had done 1000 trials of that small size. As before, he would have committed a type I error (obtained a significant P-value) in 5% of those experiments where the null hypothesis was true, but now he would have obtained a non-significant result in perhaps 75% of those trials where the effects of the two treatments differed. He would only obtain a significant P-value in 25 of the 100 trials where the alternative hypothesis was true. Consequently, he would obtain a significant P-value in 70 trials, and in 45 (64%) of these trials the null hypothesis would be true. In other words, if the sample size was that small, we should only be 34% confident that there was a difference between the treatment effects when he obtained a statistically significant P-value.

Statistical tests

The discussion so far has been concerned with the testing of hypotheses in general, but critical readers also need some knowledge of the assumptions and interpretation of the most common significance tests. We shall mention some of those that are used to compare two groups of patients, and it will be seen that the choice of test depends on the scale of measurement of the observations.

Fisher's exact test (or possibly a χ^2 test) is used to compare two rates, i.e. observations on a *binary scale*. This would be the correct choice if we wished to compare the rate of ophthalmopathy in two groups of patients.

Table 17 Dr N's research career, if the sample size had been smaller.

		Truth		
		H_A	H_0	Total
Result of significance test	P ≤ 0.05	25	45	70
	P > 0.05	75	855	930
	Total	100	900	1000

Chapter 8

The two-sample rank sum test (Mann–Whitney U-test) is used to compare two distributions of *ordinal scale* measurements. It would be the ideal test for comparing the distribution of Dr N's clinical index in two samples. The rank sum test may, however, also be used to test distributions of interval scale measurements as it is always permissible to reduce the level of measurement. It has been shown that the loss of information by doing so is minimal. Therefore, for example, the serum thyroxine concentrations in two samples may be compared using this test.

The two-sample t-test (student t-test) is used to compare two distributions of *interval scale* measurements, on the assumption that the underlying distributions are approximately Gaussian and that they have the same standard deviation. The test is robust to violation of the Gaussian assumption if the sample is large, the standard deviations similar, and the distributions not too asymmetrical, but it must not be used if the sample is small and the distribution skew. Then the two-sample rank sum test is to be preferred.

Some tests are specially suited to the analysis of cross-over trials where the observations are paired, e.g. the sign test (or McNemar test), one-sample rank sum test (Wilcoxon test), and one-sample t-test. The assumptions are those already mentioned for the two-sample tests.

The following examples illustrate some problems frequently encountered in medical papers.

In a randomized trial, cure was reported in 15 of 23 patients receiving treatment A, and in 15 of 29 patients receiving treatment B (Fisher's exact test, P > 0.20). Thus, there was no difference between the effects of the two treatments. The choice of test was correct, but the conclusion wrong. The therapeutic gain was $65\% - 52\% = 13\%$ and, using the formula on p. 136, it will be found that the 95% confidence interval of the therapeutic gain is $13 \pm 27\%$. Therefore, from a statistical point of view, it is possible that treatment A cured between 40% more patients and 14% fewer patients than treatment B.

A rating scale (with seven categories) was used to grade the patients' symptoms. The mean score was 1.61 (2 SD 1.40) in the first group and 1.90 (2 SD 1.36) in the second group. The difference is statistically significant (two-sample t-test, P < 0.05). Examples like this one are frequently found even in well-reputed medical journals. We are dealing with data measured on an ordinal scale, and statistical calculations which assume an interval scale and a Gaussian distribution are meaningless. The author should have used a two-sample rank sum test which might well have shown that the difference was non-significant.

Forty-two patients with disease A and 21 patients with disease B were compared. The mean VLDL-concentration was 346 mg/L (SE 66 mg/L) in group A and 627 mg/L (SE 93 mg/L) in group B, the difference being statistically significant (P < 0.01, two-sample t-test). In this case the observations were measured on an interval scale, but it is easy to see that the Gaussian assumption was not fulfilled. As explained on p. 186 it is possible to calculate 'backwards' from SE to SD. In group *B*, SD = $93 \times \sqrt{21}$ = 426 mg/L and, consequently, the interval mean ± 2 SD is 627 ± 852 mg/L. This calculation suggests that some of the patients had a negative VLDL-concentration which, of course, is impossible. The distribution was very skew and the sample small, so the two-sample rank sum test should have been used instead of the *t*-test. It might, however, have been permissible to use the *t*-test, if the sample had been much larger (at least 100 patients in each group), but in this case the two-sample rank sum test must be used instead.

Simvastatin treatment for 5½ years reduced the death rate from all causes by 30. This is a quotation from a Danish drug directory (commonly used by doctors in that country) and it describes correctly the results of the Scandinavian Simvastatin Survival Study [190], which was done to test the preventive effect of simvastatin in patients with ischaemic heart disease and hypercholesterolaemia. The relative risk of death (see p. 136), comparing the treatment group and the control group, was 0.71. This reduction of the death rate seems impressive, but the decision whether or not to use the treatment also depends on the absolute risk reduction, i.e. the therapeutic gain, and that information was not provided in the directory. The original paper states that 11.5% of 2223 patients in the control group died, compared with 8.2% of 2221 patients in the treatment group. Therefore, the therapeutic gain was 3.3% (95% confidence interval: 2.4%−4.2%). One might also have calculated NNT, i.e. the number of patients one needs to treat for 5½ years in order to save one life, which in this case is 1/0.033 = 30 (p. 136). That kind of information is needed to assess, among other things, the economical consequences of introducing the treatment. It has been shown that the presentation of the results of clinical studies influences the reader's assessment of the efficiency of a treatment [191].

In a large trial (almost 4000 patients), comparing clofibrate and placebo, the death rates in the two groups were almost identical (20.0% and 20.9%). However, a subgroup analysis revealed that the death rate was considerably reduced among those persons in the clofibrate group who had taken at least 80% of the prescribed medicine [192]. That result suggested that clofibrate had an effect after all. Further analysis, however, revealed that this conclusion was too hasty, as the death rate was reduced to the same extent among those persons in the control group who had taken at least 80% of their inactive tablets. The example illustrates the danger of subgroup analyses. The results of this trial only suggest that those who comply with the requirements of the protocol fare better than those who do not, regardless of the content of the tablets.

Treatment A and treatment B were compared in a randomized clinical trial. A comparison of the patients' condition before treatment and after treatment revealed that those who received treatment A presented a significant improvement (one-sample rank sum test, P < 0.05) whereas those who received treatment B did not improve significantly (NS). The author of this paper asked the question whether the condition, in each treatment group, improved during the treatment period, and it is correct to use the one-sample rank sum test to answer this question, but the question is irrelevant. He did the trial to find out whether one treatment was better than the other, but these tests do not compare the treatment results. It is quite possible that the improvement in group *A* was just statistically significant (e.g. $P = 0.04$) and in group *B* just statistically non-significant (e.g. $P = 0.06$), and such a difference may easily arise by chance. Instead the treatment results in the two groups should have been compared by means of a two-sample test. The example also shows that it is best always to state the exact *P*-value, and the expression NS should never be used. It is important to know whether the *P*-value was, say, 0.06 or 0.30.

Twenty-one (57%) of 37 patients who received treatment A were cured compared with 13 (34%) of 38 patients who received treatment B. Treatment A was found to be significantly more effective than treatment B (one-tailed Fisher's test, P = 0.04). This example illustrates a problem which we have not yet mentioned. On p. 132 the *P*-value was defined as the probability of obtaining, by chance, a difference between the treatment results which numerically is as large as (or larger than) the one observed in the study. In this case the therapeutic gain was 57%–34% = 23%, and, consequently, we expect the *P*-value to tell us the probability of obtaining a difference of at least 23%, *either* in favour of treatment *A or* in favour of treatment *B*, if the null hypothesis is true. This conventional *P*-value, which does not take into account the direction of the difference, is said to be two-sided or *two-tailed*. In this case, however, the author calculated the *one-tailed P*-value which is the probability of obtaining a difference of 23% or more in favour of treatment *A*, i.e. he ignored the possibility that treatment *A* might be less effective than *B*. From a practical point of view there is no problem. The reader should just multiply the *P*-value by two. In this case the conventional two-tailed P (sometimes called 2P) is 0.08, and the difference was statistically non-significant.

Sometimes authors use one-tailed tests (halve their *P*-values) without mentioning that they have done so and that practice borders on fraud.

A MEDLINE search was done to retrieve all randomized trials that compared the results of thrombolytic treatment with placebo or no treatment in patients who had suffered a stroke. Only papers written in English were included. Statements of this kind in reports of meta-analyses are quite common, and the reader should not accept the result without reservations. It is unacceptable that papers written in languages other than English are not included. For instance, some good trials of patients suffering from stroke have only been published in Japanese and they must not be ignored in a meta-analysis. Further, it was not stated how the MEDLINE search was done (see p. 139). The reliability of a meta-analysis depends on the thoroughness of the search, and the strategy used must be described in detail in the report.

Correlation analysis

Medical papers also report other types of statistical analyses. They may contain diagrams like Fig. 19b, which shows the correlation between the serum

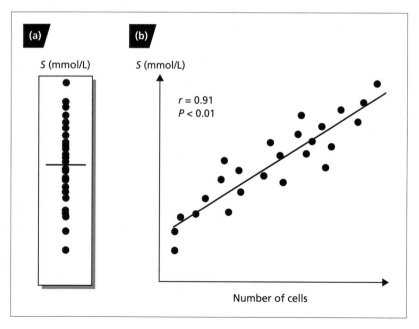

Fig. 19 (a) The serum concentration of substance *S* in 25 patients. (b) The correlation between the serum concentration of *S* and the number of a particular kind of cell in biopsy specimens from the same patients.

concentration of a substance S in 25 persons and the number of cells of a particular type in tissue specimens from the same persons. It is seen that the correlation is positive, as those patients who have a high content of S also tend to possess a large number of the cells in question. Usually a straight line, the *regression line*, is shown in such a diagram, and often the value of r, the *correlation coefficient*, and a P-value are quoted. It is the purpose of this presentation to explain the interpretation of these terms.

The researcher who did this study suspected that S was produced by a certain type of cell; he had noticed that the concentration of S varied from patient to patient (Fig. 19a), and he wanted to find out to what extent this variation could be explained by the fact that some patients possessed more cells of that particular type than others.

The favoured statistical measure of the dispersion of a series of observations is the variation around the mean, or $\Sigma(d^2)$, where, in this case, d is the difference between the concentration of S in the individual patient and the mean concentration of S in the whole sample. Therefore, in principle, the researcher measured the vertical distances between the individual points and the mean in Fig. 19a, squared these distances and calculated the sum. In correlation analysis this sum is called the *total variation* (or simply the sum of squares).

Next, as shown in Fig. 19b, the researcher related the concentrations of S to the number of cells in each patient, and, in order to interpret that relationship, he once again determined the variation of S, only this time he calculated the variation around the regression line, i.e. in principle, he measured the vertical distances between the points and the line, squared those distances and calculated the sum. This sum is called the residual variation. The regression line has been constructed in such a way that the *residual variation* around that line is smaller than the variation around any other line.

It is seen at a glance that the residual variation (the variation around the line) is much smaller than the total variation (the variation around the mean), which means that part of the variation in the concentration of S is explained by the variation in the number of cells in the patients in question. The *explained variation* is the difference between the total and the residual variation.

The meaning of this terminology is grasped most easily by considering two extremes, perfect correlation and no correlation at all. If the correlation had been perfect, all the points in Fig. 19b would have been situated on the regression line, and the residual variation would have been zero, meaning that the total variation had been fully explained. If, on the other hand, there had been no correlation, the points would have been evenly scattered, and the regression line would have been horizontal (on the level of the mean concentration of S). The residual variation would have been identical with the total variation, and nothing would have been explained.

The correlation coefficient, r, or the *determination coefficient*, r^2, are used to indicate the strength of the correlation. Usually, r is quoted, but r^2 is easier to interpret, as shown by this formula:

$$r^2 = \frac{explained\ variation}{total\ variation}$$

In our example, $r = 0.91$ and consequently $r^2 = 0.83$. This means that the explained variation is 83% of the total variation, i.e. that 83% of the variation in the concentration of S is explained by the fact that some patients have more cells of the particular type than others. The residual variation is only 17% of the total variation around the mean in Fig. 19a. The word 'explained' in these examples must, of course, not be taken at face value, as a positive or negative correlation between the y- and x-values does not necessarily imply that the variation of y is caused by the variation of x. It is also possible that the variation of x is caused by that of y or that both variations have a common cause.

In this example, the correlation was positive, and r was positive. The correlation may also be negative (the larger the value of x, the smaller the value of y), and in that case r would be negative. Thus the correlation coefficient varies from -1 (perfect negative correlation), over zero (no correlation), to $+1$ (perfect positive correlation).

The correlation coefficient is a numerical characteristic of that particular sample, and as such it is subject to random variation. It may be larger or smaller than the 'true' correlation coefficient of the population, and therefore it is necessary to consider the possibility that the truth is that there is no correlation at all. This possibility is tested by a special significance test. In the example $r = 0.91$ and $P < 0.01$, which means that there is less than a one per cent chance of obtaining an r-value which differs that much from zero if in fact there is no correlation at all. It is also possible to calculate the 95% confidence intervals of r and r^2.

Conventional correlation analysis assumes that the measurements have been recorded on an interval scale and that both the x-values and the y-values form a Gaussian distribution. If these assumptions are not fulfilled, it is necessary to use a ranking method, such as a *Spearman test*, and to calculate a rank correlation coefficient (R_s), which is tested against zero just like the conventional correlation coefficient. R_s and r are almost identical, if the distribution is Gaussian.

The following examples illustrate some of those hazards of correlation analyses which are frequently ignored by clinical researchers.

A strong negative correlation was found between the gastric acid production and the age in a sample of 250 men with duodenal ulcer (P < 0.0001). These authors mistakenly believed that the correlation is strong when the P-value is small. In this case, $r = -0.56$ and $r^2 = 0.31$ which means that the correlation was quite weak. Only 31% of the variation in acid production is explained by the age variation. However, the author had studied so many patients that it is extremely unlikely that this weak correlation was a chance finding.

The clinical index in 80 patients and the collagen content of their liver biopsies showed a significant positive correlation (r = 0.28, P = 0.01). The data and the regression line are shown in Fig. 20. The assumptions of the analysis, however, were violated as the distributions of both variables were far from Gaussian and, in addition, the clinical index is not measured on an interval scale, but on an ordinal scale. In this case, the authors ought to have done a Spearman test which would have revealed that the P-value was 0.20.

Figure 21 shows the correlation between the serum concentrations of two

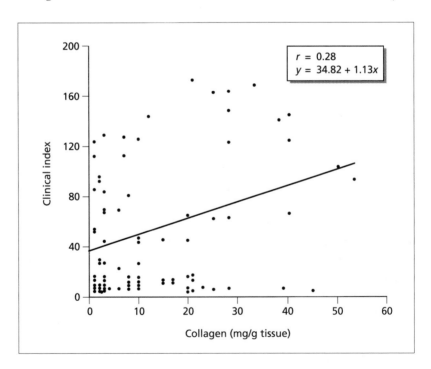

Fig. 20 The correlation between a clinical index and the collagen content of biopsies from 80 patients with a particular disease.

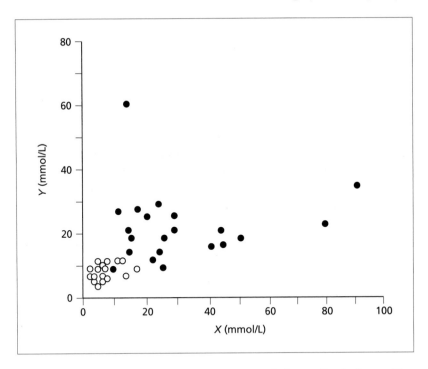

Fig. 21 The correlation between the serum concentrations of substance *X* and substance *Y* in 17 healthy subjects (open circle;) and 21 patients with a particular disease (black circle).

substances, Y and X. A Spearman test gave the result $R_S = 0.71$, *P<0.001.* In this case the choice of test presented no problem, but in spite of that the analysis made little sense. The text shows that we are not dealing with one sample of 38 persons, but with two samples: 17 normal controls and 21 patients suffering from a particular disease. If we look at each of these samples in isolation, there is no obvious correlation between *X* and *Y*. The positive correlation only appears when we combine the samples, and that is impermissible. This is sometimes called the 'mouse–elephant' phenomenon. There is probably no positive correlation between the age and length of adult mice, nor between the age and length of adult elephants, but if we analysed a combined sample of 50 mice and 50 elephants, we should obtain a highly significant positive correlation and a minute *P*-value. There would be 50 points in the lower left corner and 50 in the upper right corner of the coordinate system.

Life table analysis

Five hundred and twelve patients with a particular type of leukaemia were

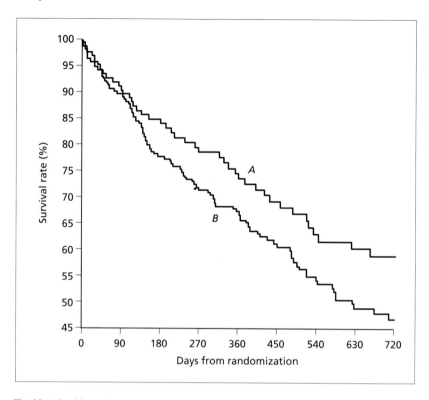

Fig. 22 Life table graph (Kaplan–Maier plot) illustrating the results of a randomized clinical trial.

allocated at random to treatment A or treatment B. The Kaplan–Maier plots
(Fig. 22) show that the patients receiving treatment A fared better than those
receiving treatment B (logrank test: P = 0.02). The cumulative two-year survival rate was 58% in group A and 46% in group B. Each 'step' on the graphs
(which are often called Kaplan–Maier plots) represents the death of one
patient, and they illustrate well the results of this trial. The simplicity of the
illustration, however, is somewhat deceptive. The critical reader of this paper
might notice that the trial ran from 1 January 1996 to 30 June 1998, during
which period all patients fulfilling the entry criteria were admitted and seen
regularly. On the latter date the trial closed, and no more observations were
made. Consequently, those patients who were admitted within the last year of
the trial period were observed for less than two years. How then is it possible
to calculate the two-year survival rate?

This type of analysis is very useful and therefore we shall explain the
basic principles [7,193,194]. Imagine a small prognostic study which aims at
estimating the one-year survival rate of patients suffering from a particular

disease. The trial period was 18 months (1 Jan. 1997 to 30 June 1998) and during that period of time seven patients with this disease were seen. The crude observations are shown in Table 18a. It is seen that the first patient was observed for more than one year before the closing date (30 June 1998). The fifth and the sixth patients were also alive on the closing date, but had been observed for less than one year. The remaining four patients died during the study. In Table 18b this information has been reorganized. The day of entry for all patients has been called day 1 and the patients have been ranked according to the observation time. Now we may regard this sample as a small cohort of patients who all entered the study on the same day, but were observed for varying periods of time until they died or until the closure of the trial.

The statistician then calculates the survival rate whenever one of the patients leaves the cohort. On day 101 one patient died which means that the survival rate that day was 6/7 or 0.86. On day 146 one of the remaining six patients died, meaning that the survival rate that day was $5/6 = 0.83$. On day 193 one of the remaining 5 patients was lost to the cohort, but he was still alive so the survival rate on that day was 1. Now only 4 patients were left, and, consequently, the survival rate on day 254 when one of them died was

Table 18 Life table from a small prognostic study. (a) The crude data from a small prognostic single-cohort study of seven patients. (b) The day of entry for all patients has been labelled day 1. The patients have been listed according to the length of the observation time.

Patient No.	Date of entry	Date of exit	Status at exit
(a)			
1	21.1.97	30.6.98	Still alive
2	20.1.97	1.10.97	Died
3	12.5.97	16.2.98	Died
4	24.6.97	3.10.97	Died
5	12.10.97	30.6.98	Still alive
6	19.12.97	30.6.98	Still alive
7	5.1.98	31.5.98	Died
(b)			
4	1	101	Died
7	1	146	Died
5	1	193	Still alive
2	1	254	Died
6	1	261	Still alive
3	1	280	Died
1	1	525	Still alive

only 3/4 = 0.75. On day 261 one of the remaining three patients was lost to follow-up, leaving two, which means that the survival rate on day 280 when one patient died was only 50%. The last patient survived until the trial closed.

Next, the statistician calculates the successive cumulative survival rates. The chance that a patient entering the trial on day one will survive day 101 and 146 is $0.86 \times 0.83 = 0.71$, the chance that he will survive day 101, 146 and 254 is $0.86 \times 0.83 \times 0.75 = 0.54$, and the chance that he will also survive day 280 is $0.87 \times 0.83 \times 0.75 \times 0.50 = 0.27$. This is the cumulative one-year survival time. Figure 23 is a Kaplan–Maier plot which, just like Fig. 22, shows the successive reduction of the cumulative survival rate.

Patients number 5 and 6 illustrate well the advantage of these rather cumbersome calculations (which if the sample is large requires computer assistance). They were not observed for a full year, but they are included in the calculation until the time when they left the cohort. The cumulative one-year survival rate incorporates the information that they survived that long. In

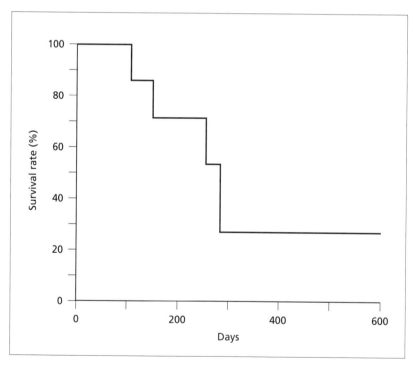

Fig. 23 Life table graph (Kaplan–Maier plot) illustrating the results of a small single-cohort prognostic study.

large studies there are many such patients, and their inclusion may greatly influence the end result.

It is possible to calculate the 95% confidence interval of the cumulative survival rate [195], and it is also possible to compare the survival of two cohorts by means of a special significance test, the so-called logrank test. This was done in the example illustrated by Fig. 22. It is important to note that the test does not just compare the cumulative survival rates, but the differences throughout the whole course of the study.

Life table analysis is not only used in survival studies. It is also extremely useful for the analysis of other types of events, such as recurrences of a disease (e.g. recurrent myocardial infarctions), the development of complications (e.g. cerebrovascular attacks in cohorts of hypertensive persons) or the development of metastases in patients with malignant diseases.

References

Those references which are marked with an asterisk are considered particularly useful for further studies.

Selected books

Clinical decision-making and clinical research methods

* 1 Feinstein AR. *Clinical Judgment*. Baltimore: Williams & Wilkins, 1967.
  2 Lusted LB. *Introduction to Medical Decision Making*. Springfield: CC Thomas, 1968.
  3 Galen RS, Gambino SR. *Beyond Normality: The Predictive Value and Efficiency of Medical Diagnoses*. New York: Wiley, 1975.
* 4 Feinstein AR. *Clinical Biostatistics*. Saint Louis: Mosby, 1977.
  5 Philips CI, Wolfe JN. eds. *Clinical Practice and Economics*. Tunbridge Wells: Pitman Medical, 1977.
  6 Weinstein MC, Fineberg HV. *Clinical Decision Analysis*. Philadelphia: Saunders, 1980.
* 7 Pocock SJ. *Clinical Trials. A Practical Approach*. Chichester: Wiley, 1983.
* 8 Feinstein AR. *Clinical Epidemiology. The Architecture of Clinical Research*. Philadelphia: Saunders, 1985.
* 9 Feinstein AR. *Clinimetrics*. New Haven: Yale University Press, 1987.
* 10 Sackett DL, Haynes RB, Guyatt GH *et al. Clinical Epidemiology. A Basic Science for Clinical Medicine*, 2nd edn. Boston: Little Brown, 1991.
  11 Sackett DL, Richardson WS, Rosenberg W *et al. Evidence-Based Medicine*. New York: Churchill Livingstone, 1997.

Medical statistics

  12 Hill A, Bradford A. *Short Textbook of Medical Statistics*. London: Hodder & Stoughton, 1977.
* 13 Siegel S, Castellan NJ. *Non-Parametric Statistics for the Behavioral Sciences*, 2nd edn. New York: McGraw-Hill, 1988.
* 14 Andersen B. *Methodological Errors in Medical Research*. Oxford: Blackwell Scientific Publications, 1990.

References

* 15 Fleiss JL. *Statistical Methods for Rates and Proportions*, 2nd edn. New York: Wiley, 1981.

* 16 Altman DG. *Practical Statistics for Medical Research*. London: Chapman & Hall, 1991.

* 17 Armitage P, Berry G. *Statistical Methods in Medical Research*, 3rd edn. Oxford: Blackwell Science, 1994.

Medical history

* 18 Faber K. *Nosography in Modern Internal Medicine*. London: Humphrey Milford, 1923.

19 Garrison FH. *An Introduction to the History of Medicine*, 4th edn. Philadelphia: Saunders, 1929.

20 Major RH. *Classic Descriptions of Disease*, 3rd edn. Springfield: CC Thomas, 1945.

21 Lasagna L. *The Doctor's Dilemmas*. London: Gollancz, 1962.

22 Clendening L. *Source Book of Medical History*. New York: Dover, 1960.

* 23 Conrad LI, Neve M, Nutton V *et al*. *The Western Medical Tradition 800 BC to AD 1800*. Cambridge: Cambridge University Press, 1995.

Medical philosophy

* 24 Murphy EA. *The Logic of Medicine*. Baltimore: Johns Hopkins University Press, 1976.

* 25 Wulff HR, Pedersen SA, Rosenberg R. *Philosophy of Medicine*, 2nd edn. Oxford: Blackwell Scientific Publications, 1990.

Medical ethics

* 26 Beauchamp TL. *Philosophical Ethics. An Introduction to Moral Philosophy*, 2nd edn. New York: McGraw-Hill, 1991.

* 27 BMAs Ethics, Science & Information Division. *Medical Ethics Today: Its Practice and Philosophy*. London: BMJ Publishing Group, 1993.

28 Gillon R, ed. *Principles of Health Care Ethics*. Chichester: Wiley, 1993.

Other references

29 Wulff HR, Andersen B, Brandenhoff P *et al*. What do doctors know about statistics? *Stat Med* 1987; 6: 3–10.

30 Lindley D. *Making Decisions*. London: Wiley-Interscience, 1971.

31 Harpestreng H. *Liber Herbarum*. (13th Century, in Latin and Danish.) (ed. P Hauberg) Copenhagen: Hafnia, 1936.

32 Stevens S. On the theory of scales of measurement. *Science* 1946; 103: 677–80.

33 Huskisson EC. Measurement of pain. *Lancet* 1974; ii: 1127–31.

34 Gøtzsche PC. Sensitivity of effect variables in rheumatoid arthritis: a meta-analysis of 130 placebo controlled NSAID trials. *J Clin Epidemiol* 1990; 43: 1313–8.

35 Cit. in ref. 9, p. 9.

36 Apgar V, Holiday DA, James S *et al*. Evaluation of the newborn infant. *JAMA* 1958; 168: 1985–8.

37 Knaus WA, Draper EA, Wagner DP *et al*. APACHE II – a severity of disease classification system. *Crit Care Med* 1985; 13: 818–29.

38 Gøtzsche PC. Methodology and overt and hidden bias in reports of 196 double-blind trials of nonsteroidal, antiinflammatory drugs in rheumatoid arthritis. *Controlled Clin Trials* 1989; 10: 31–56 (erratum: 356).

39 Higgins ITT, Cochrane AL, Thomas AJ. Epidemiological studies of coronary disease. *Br J Prev Soc Med* 1963; 17: 153–65.

40 Anonymous. Why did I ask for this pathological investigation? *Lancet* 1957; ii: 890.

41 Hansen UM. Oral temperaturmåling. (English summary.) *Ugeskr Læger* 1991; 153: 3535–7.

42 Christensen PM, Christensen VB, Matzen LE. Evaluering af øretemperatur-måling på en geriatrisk afdeling. (English summary.) *Ugeskr Læger* 1998; 160: 5175–7.

43 Garland LH. Studies on the accuracy of diagnostic procedures. *Am J Roentgenol* 1959; 82: 25–8.

44 Yerushalmy J, Harkness JT, Cope JH *et al*. The role of dual reading in mass radiography. *Am Rev Tub* 1950; 61: 443–63.

45 Spitzer RL, Cohen J, Fleiss JL *et al*. Quantification of agreement in psychiatric diagnosis: a new approach. *Arch Gen Psychiatry* 1967; 17: 83–7.

46 Koran LM. The reliability of clinical methods, data and judgments. *N Engl J Med* 1975; 293: 642–6 and 695–701.

47 Herlev Hospital Study Group. Diagnostic decision process in suspected pulmonary embolism. *Lancet* 1979; i: 1336–8.

48 Feinstein AR, Cicchetti DV. High agreement but low kappa. I and II. *J Clin Epidemiol* 1990; 43: 543–50 and 551–8.

49 Feinstein AR. A bibliography of publications on observer variability. *J Chron Dis* 1985; 38: 619–32.

50 Gjørup T, Agner E, Jensen LB *et al*. The endoscopic diagnosis of gastric ulcer. A randomized clinical trial of interobserver variation and bias induced by knowledge of the radiological diagnosis. *Scand J Gastroenterol* 1985; 20: 554–8.

51 Gjørup T, Agner E, Jensen LB *et al*. The endoscopic diagnosis of duodenal ulcer disease. A randomized clinical trial of bias and interobserver variation. *Scand J Gastroenterol* 1986; 21: 561–7.

52 Gjørup T, Bugge PM, Jensen AM. Interobserver variation in assessment of respiratory signs. *Acta Med Scand* 1984; 216: 61–6.

53 Gjørup T, Bugge PM, Hendriksen C *et al*. A critical evaluation of the clinical diagnosis of anemia. *Am J Epidemiol* 1986; 124: 657–65.

References

54 Frisch T, Simonsen L, Hilden J. Observatørvariation og akkuratesse ved klinisk ascitesbedømmelse. (English summary.) *Ugeskr Læger* 1991; 153: 1864–8.

55 Korsgaard B, Marcussen H, Wulff HR *et al*. Den udvidede histaminprøve som diagnostisk hjælpemiddel. (English summary.) *Ugeskr Læger* 1968; 130: 1657–64.

56 Pilgaard S, Krag E, Wulff HR. Rutinemæssig thoraxrøntgenundersøgelse og elektrokardiografi i et gastroenterologisk forambulatorium. (English summary.) *Ugeskr Læger* 1975; 137: 2817–20.

57 The Swedish Council on Technology Assessment in Health Care (SBU). *Preoperative Routines*. Stockholm: SBU, 1989.

58 Winkens RAG, Pop P, Grol RPTM *et al*. Effects of routine individual feedback over nine years on general practitioners' requests for tests. *BMJ* 1996; 312: 490.

59 Riggs BL, Hodgson SF, O'Fallon WM *et al*. Effect of fluoride treatment on the fracture rate in postmenopausal women with osteoporosis. *N Engl J Med* 1990; 322: 802–9.

60 Jones FA ed. *Richard Asher Talking Sense*. London: Pitman Medical, 1972.

61 Faber K. Historical outline of medical therapy. In: Faber K. *Lectures on Internal Medicine*. New York: Hoeber, 1927.

62 Gotfredsen E. *Medicinens Historie*. (In Danish.) Copenhagen: Busck, 1950.

63 Cit. in ref. 19, p. 288.

64 Campbell EJM. The science of diagnosis. In: Philips CI, Wolfe JN. eds. *Clinical Practice and Economics*. Tunbridge Wells: Pitman Medical, 1977; 101–12.

65 Prigogine I, Stengers I. *Order Out of Chaos*. Toronto: Bantam, 1984.

66 Stewart I. *Does God Play Dice?* Harmondsworth: Penguin, 1989.

67 Cohen J, Stewart I. *The Collapse of Chaos*. New York: Penguin, 1995.

68 Pedersen SA. Disease entities and open systems. In: Querido A, van Es LA, Mandema E. eds. *The Discipline of Medicine. Emerging Concepts and Their Impact on Medical Research and Medical Education*. Amsterdam: North Holland, 1984.

69 Goodwin B. *How the Leopard Changed its Spots. The Evolution of Complexity*. London: Phoenix, 1994.

70 Barker DJP. *Mothers, Babies and Disease in Later Life*. London: BMJ Publishing Group, 1994.

71 Goldberger AL, Rigney DR, West BJ. Chaos and fractals in human physiology. *Scientific American* 1990; Febr: 35–90.

72 Goldberger AL. Non-linear dynamics for clinicians: chaos theory, fractals, and complexity at the bedside. *Lancet* 1996; 347: 312–4.

73 Weiss JN, Garfinkel A, Spano ML, Ditto WL. Chaos and chaos control in biology. *J Clin Invest* 1994; 93: 1355–60.

74 Kanters JK, Højgaard MV, Agner E, Holstein-Rathlou N-E. Short- and long-term variation in non-linear dynamics of heart rate variability. *Cardiovasc Res* 1996; 31: 400–9.

75 Holstein-Rathlou N-H, Marsh DJ. Renal blood flow regulation and arterial pressure regulations: a case study of nonlinear dynamics. *Physiol Rev* 1994; 3: 637–81.

76 Pool R. Is it healthy to be chaotic? *Science* 1989; 241: 604–7.

77 Nesse RM, Williams GC, Evolution, Healing. *The New Science of Darwinian Medicine*. London: Phoenix, 1996.

78 McKeown T. *The Origins of Human Disease*. Oxford: Basil Blackwell, 1988.

79 With C. *Mavesaarets kliniske Former, dets Diagnose og Behandling.* (In Danish.) Copenhagen: Gyldendal, 1881.

80 Jennings D. Perforated peptic ulcer. Changes Age-Incidence Sex-Distribution Last 150 Years. *Lancet* 1940; i: 395–8 and 444–7.

81 Kendell RE. *The Role of Diagnosis in Psychiatry*. Oxford: Blackwell Scientific Publications, 1975; 72.

82 Riis P, Anthonisen P. The differential diagnosis between ulcerative colitis and Crohn's disease of the colon. In: Gregor O, Riedl O. eds. *Modern Gastroenterology*. Stuttgart: Schattauer, 1969; 912.

83 Lipsky PE. Rheumatoid arthritis. In: Fauci SA *et al.* eds. *Harrison's Principles of Internal Medicine,* 14th edn. New York: McGraw-Hill, 1998; 1885.

84 Mackie JL. *The Cement of the Universe. A Study of Causation*. London: Oxford University Press, 1974.

85 Zeta (pseudonym). *The Diagnosis of the Acute Abdomen in Rhyme*. London: H. K. Lewis, 1955.

86 Puylaert JBCM, Rutgers PH, Lalisang RI *et al.* A prospective study of ultrasonography in the diagnosis of appendicitis. *N Engl J Med* 1987; 317: 666–9.

87 Johnsen R, Bernersen B, Straume B *et al.* Prevalences of endoscopic and histological findings in subjects with and without dyspepsia. *BMJ* 1991; 302: 749–52.

88 Horvath WJ. The effect of physician bias in medical diagnosis. *Behav Sci* 1964; 9: 334–40.

89 Grande P, Christiansen C, Pedersen A, Christensen MS. Rationel diagnostik ved akut myokardieinfarkt. (English summary.) *Ugeskr Læger* 1980; 142: 1565–9.

90 Harvey RF. Indices of thyroid function in thyrotoxicosis. *Lancet* 1971; ii: 230–3.

91 Cobb S. On the development of diagnostic criteria. *Arthritis Rheum* 1960; 3: 91–5.

92 Reid MC, Mark SL, Feinstein AR. Use of methodological standards in diagnostic test research. *JAMA* 1995; 274: 645–51.

93 Schmidt WA, Kraft HE, Vorpahl K *et al.* Color duplex ultrasonography in the diagnosis of temporal arteritis. *N Engl J Med* 1997; 337: 1336–42.

94 Meador CK. Non-disease: a problem of overdiagnosis. *Diagnostica (Ames Corp)* 1969; 3: 10–11.

95 Meador CK. The art and science of non-disease. *N Eng J Med* 1965; 272: 92–5.

96 Bull JP. The historical development of clinical therapeutic trials. *J Chron Dis* 1959; 10: 218–48.

97 Huxham J. A method for preserving the health of seamen in long cruises and voyages. 1747; Cit. In Ref., 19; 592–3.

98 Withering W *An Account of the Foxglove and Some of its Medical Uses*. Birminghan: Swinney, 1785; Cit. in: Garrison FH. *An Introduction to the History of Medicine*, 4th edn. Philadelphia: Saunders, 1929; 440–1.

99 Cit. in ref. 22; 192–3.

References

100 Gavaret J. *Principes Généraux de Statistique Médicale*. (Quoted from Danish translation.) Copenhagen: Reitzel, 1840.

101 Fenger CE. Om den numeriske Methode. (In Danish.) *Ugeskr Læger* 1839; 1: 305–15 and 321–5.

102 Louis PCA. *Recherches sur les Effets de la Saignée dans Quelques Maladies Inflammatoires*. Paris: Baillères, 1835.

103 Löwy I. *The Polish School of Philosophy of Medicine*. Philosophy of Medicine Series, No 39. Dordrect: Kluwer, 1990.

104 Bieganski W. *Medizinische Logik*. (Translated from Polish.) Würzburg: Curt Kaubitzsch, 1909.

105 Kaye MD, Rhodes J, Beck P *et al*. A controlled trial of glycopyrronium and l-hyoscyamine in the long-term treatment of duodenal ulcer. *Gut* 1970; 11: 559–66.

106 Anonymous. Anticholinergics, duodenal ulcer. *Lancet* 1970; ii: 1173.

107 Sturdevant RAL, Isenberg JI, Secrist D *et al*. Antacid and placebo produced similar relief in duodenal ulcer patients. *Gastroenterology* 1977; 72: 1–5.

108 Peterson WI, Sturdevant RAL, Frankl HD *et al*. Healing of duodenal ulcer with an antacid regimen. *N Engl J Med* 1977; 297: 341–5.

109 Jacobsen. Belladonna mod kighoste. (In Danish.) *Bibliotek Læger* 1809; 1: 105–6.

110 Williams SGJ, Westaby D. Management of variceal haemorrhage. *BMJ* 1994; 308: 1213–7.

111 Bornman PC, Krige JEJ, Terblanche J. Management of oesophageal varices. *Lancet* 1994; 343: 1079–84.

112 Galton F. Regression towards mediocrity in hereditary stature. *J Anthropol Instit Great Britain Ireland* 1885; 15: 246–63.

113 Lentner C. ed. *Geigy Scientific Tables*, Vol. 2, 8th edn. Basel: Ciba-Geigy, 1982.

114 Hróbjartsson A. *The placebo effect – a therapeutical phenomenon between science and humanities, body and mind*. M.Phil. Thesis, Glasgow University, 1993.

115 Gøtzsche PC. Is there logic in the placebo? *Lancet* 1994; 344: 925–6.

116 Grünbaum A. The placebo concept in medicine and psychiatry. *Psychol Med* 1986; 16: 19–38.

117 Brody H. *Placebos and the Philosophy of Medicine*. Chicago: University of Chicago Press, 1980.

118 Kienle GS, Kiene H. Placebo effect and placebo concept: a critical methodological and conceptual analysis of reports on the magnitude of the placebo effect. *Forschende Komplementärmedizin* 1996; 3: 121–38.

119 Beecher HK. The powerful placebo. *JAMA* 1955; 159: 1602–6.

120 Kleijnen J, de Craen AJM, van Everdingen J *et al*. Placebo effect in double-blind clinical trials: a review of interactions with medications. *Lancet* 1994; 344: 1347–9.

121 Thomas KB. General practice consultations: is there any point in being positive? *BMJ* 1987; 284: 1200–2.

122 Hodnett ED. Support from caregivers during childbirth. In: The Cochrane Library (disk & CD-ROM). Oxford: Update Software, 1996.

123 Hróbjartsson A, Gøtzsche PC, Gluud C. The controlled clinical trial turns 100 years: Fibiger's trial of serum treatment of diphtheria. *BMJ* 1998; 317: 1243–5.

124 Medical Research Council. Streptomycin treatment of pulmonary tuberculosis. *BMJ* 1948; 2: 769–82.

125 Saunders J. Alternative, complementary, holistic . . . In: Greaves D, Upton H. *Philosophical Problems in Health Care*. Avebury: Avebury, 1996: 103–25.

126 Salmon JW. Ed. *Alternative Medicines*. London: Tavistock,1985; 67.

127 Coulter HL. Homoeopathy. In: Salmon JW. ed. *Alternative Medicines*. London: Tavistock, 1985.

128 Caplan RL. Chiropractic. In: Salmon JW. ed. *Alternative Medicines*. London: Tavistock, 1985.

129 Meade TW, Dyer S, Browne W *et al*. Low back pain of mechanical origin: randomised comparison of chiropractic and hospital outpatient treatment. *BMJ* 1990; 300: 1431–7.

130 Mostefa-Kara N, Pauwels A, Pines E *et al*. Fatal hepatitis after herbal tea. (Letter.) *Lancet* 1992; 340: 674.

131 Popper KR. *Conjectures and Refutations*. 5th edn. London: Routledge and Kegan Paul, 1974.

132 Linde K, Clausius N, Ramirez G *et al*. Are the clinical effects of homoeopathy placebo effects? A meta-analysis of placebo-controlled trials. *Lancet* 1997; 350: 834–43.

133 Bernard CL. *Introduction à l'Étude de la Médicine Expérimentale*. 1866; Reprinted London: Garnier-Flammarion, 1966.

134 Schulz KF, Chalmers I, Hayes RJ *et al*. Empirical evidence of bias: dimensions of methodological quality associated with estimates of treatment effects in controlled trials. *JAMA* 1995; 273: 408–12.

135 Majeed AW, Troy G, Nicholl JP *et al*. Randomised prospective, single-blind comparison of laparoscopic versus small-incision cholecystectomy. *Lancet* 1996; 347: 989–94.

136 Gøtzsche PC, Liberati A, Luca P *et al*. Beware of surrogate outcome measures. *Int J Technol Assessment Health Care* 1996; 12: 238–46.

137 Psaty BM, Heckbert SR, Koepsell TD *et al*. The risk of myocardial infarction associated with antihypertensive therapies. *JAMA* 1995; 274: 620–5.

138 The Cardiac Arrhythmia Suppression Trial (CAST). Preliminary report: effect of encainide and flecainide on mortality in a randomized trial of arrhythmia suppression after myocardial infarction. *N Engl J Med* 1989; 321: 406–12.

139 Moore TJ. *Deadly Medicine*. New York: Simon and Schuster 1995.

140 McFadden ER. Asthma. In: Fauci AS *et al*. eds. *Harrison's Principles of Internal Medicine*. New York: McGraw-Hill, 1998: 1425.

141 Wulff HR. Confidence limits in evaluating controlled clinical trials. *Lancet* 1973; 2: 969–70.

142 Interpreting clinical trials. (Editorial.) *BMJ* 1978; ii: 1317.

143 Altman DG, Gore SM, Gardner MJ *et al*. Statistical Guidelines for Contributors to Medical Journals. *BMJ* 1983; 286: 1489–93.

144 In ref. 10: 205–9.

References

145 Yusuf S, Wittes J, Probstfield J *et al*. Analysis and interpretation of treatment effects in subgroups of patients in randomized clinical trials. *JAMA* 1991; 266: 93–8.

146 ISIS-2 Collaborative Group. Randomised trial of intravenous streptokinase, oral aspirin, both, or neither among 17 187 cases of suspected acute myocardial infarction: ISIS–2. *Lancet* 1988; ii: 349–60.

147 Dickersin K, Min Y-I. NIH clinical trials and publication bias. *Online J Curr Clin Trials* 1993; April 28; Doc No 50.

148 Egger M, Smith GD. Meta-analysis bias in location and selection of studies. *BMJ* 1998; 316: 61–6.

149 Mulrow CD, Oxman AD, eds. *Cochrane Collaboration Handbook*. In: The Cochrane Library (disk & CD-ROM). Oxford: Update Software, 1996.

* 150 Gøtzsche PC. Bias in double-blind trials. (Thesis.) *Dan Med Bull* 1990; 37: 329–36.

151 Begg C, Eastwood S, Horton R *et al*. Improving the quality of reporting randomized controlled trials. The CONSORT Statement. *JAMA* 1996; 276: 637–9.

152 Chalmers I, Altman DG, eds. *Systematic Reviews*. London: BMJ Publishing Group, 1995.

153 The Cochrane Library (disk & CD-ROM). The Cochrane Collaboration; Oxford: Update Software, 1996. (Updated quarterly.)

154 Gifford RH, Feinstein AR. A critique of methodology in studies of anticoagulant therapy for acute myocardial infarction. *N Engl J Med* 1969; 280: 351–7.

155 Moher D, Pham B, Jones A *et al*. Does quality of reports of randomised trials affect estimates of intervention efficacy reported in meta-analyses? *Lancet* 1998; 352: 609–13.

156 Antman EM, Lau J, Kupelnick B *et al*. A comparison of results of meta-analyses of randomized control trials and recommendations of clinical experts: treatments for myocardial infarction. *JAMA* 1992; 268: 240–8.

157 Crowley P. Corticosteroids prior to preterm delivery. In: The Cochrane Library (disk & CD-ROM). Oxford: Update Software, 1996.

158 Berlin JA, Begg CB, Louis TA. An assessment of publication bias using a sample of published clinical trials. *J Am Stat Ass* 1989; 84: 381–92.

159 Gilbert JP, McPeek B, Mosteller F. Progress in surgery and anesthesia: benefits and risks of innovative therapy. In: Bunker JP. ed. *Costs, Risks and Benefits of Surgery*. New York: Oxford University Press, 1977: 124–69.

160 Colditz GA, Miller JN, Mosteller F. How study design affects outcomes in comparisons of therapy. I Medical. *Stat Med* 1989; 8: 441–54.

161 Miller JN, Colditz GA, Mosteller F. How study design affects outcomes in comparisons of therapy. II Surgical. *Stat Med* 1989; 8: 455–68.

162 Engel GL. Commentary. In: Odegaard CE. *Dear Doctor. A Personal Letter to a Physician*. Menlo Park: The Henry J Kaiser Family Foundation, 1986: 157.

163 Ewing AC. *Ethics*. London: English University Press, 1953: vi.

164 Kübler-Ross E. *On Death and Dying*. New York: Macmillan, 1969.

165 Lunde IM. *Patienters egenvurdering. Et perspektivskift*. (Thesis, English summary.) Copenhagen: Fadl's forlag, 1990.

166 Frøjk M. *Kronisk nyresyg*. PhD Thesis (In Danish). Odense University, 1992.

167 Denzin NK, Lincoln YS, eds. *Handbook of Qualitative Research*. Thousand Oaks: Sage, 1994.

168 Kollemorten I, Strandberg C, Thomsen BM *et al*. Ethical aspects of clinical decision-making. *J Med Ethics* 1981; 7: 67–9.

169 The Gospel according to St. Matthew; 7: 12.

170 Stanley JM. Ed. The Appleton consensus. Suggested international guidelines for decisions to forgo medical treatment. *J Med Ethics* 1989; 15: 129–36.

171 Wulff HR. Against the four principles: a Nordic view. In: BMAs Ethics, Science & Information Division. *Medical Ethics Today: Its Practice and Philosophy*. London: BMJ Publishing Group, 1993: 277–86.

172 Thomsen OØ, Wulff HR, Martin A *et al*. What do gastroenterologists in Europe tell cancer patients? *Lancet* 1993; 341: 473–6.

173 In ref. 27: 161.

174 Wulff HR. The inherent paternalism of clinical practice. *J Med Phil* 1995; 20: 299–311.

175 Anonymous. Dutch euthanasia for mental torment. *BMJ* 1994; 308: 431–2.

* 176 Declaration of Helsinki. Recommendations guiding medical doctors in biomedical research involving human subjects. In: BMAs Ethics, Science & Information Division. *Medical Ethics Today: Its Practice and Philosophy*. London: BMJ Publishing Group, 1993: 330.

177 Buchanan WW, Smythe HA. Can clinicians and statisticians be friends? *J Rheumatol* 1982; 9: 653–4.

178 Greenhalgh T. *How to Read a Paper: the Basics of Evidence Based Medicine*. London: BMJ Publishing Group, 1997.

179 Andersen P, Holm P. *Problems with P*. Basle: Editiones Roche, 1984.

180 Feinstein AR, Horwitz RI. Double standards, scientific methods, and epidemiologic research. *N Engl J Med* 1982; 307: 1611–7.

181 Gjersøe P, Andersen SE, Mølbak AG *et al*. Pålideligheden af dødsattester. (English summary.) *Ugeskrift Læger* 1998; 160: 5030–4.

182 Brind J, Chincilli VM, Severs WB *et al*. Induced abortion as an independent risk factor for breast cancer: a comprehensive review and meta-analysis. *J Epidemiol Community Health* 1996; 50: 481–96.

183 Lindefors-Harris BM, Eklund G, Adami HO *et al*. Response bias in a case-control study: analysis utilizing comparative data concerning legal abortions from two independent Swedish studies. *Am J Epidemiol* 1991; 134: 1003–8.

184 Melbye M, Wohlfahrt J, Olsen JH *et al*. Induced abortion and the risk of breast cancer. *N Engl J Med* 1997; 336: 81–5.

185 Berkson J. Limitations of the application of fourfold table analysis to hospital data. *Biomet Bull* 1946; 2: 47–53.

186 Campbell MJ, Gardner MJ. Calculating confidence intervals for some non-parametric analyses. *BMJ* 1988; 296: 1454–6.

187 Morris JA, Gardner MJ. Calculating confidence limits for relative risks (odds ratios) and standardised ratios and rates. *BMJ* 1988; 296: 1313–6.

188 McLarty DG, Webber RH, Jaatinen M *et al*. Chemoprophylaxis of malaria in non-immune residents in Dar es Salaam. *Tanzania Lancet* 1984; 2: 656–9.

References

189 Wulff HR. *Magic of P-Values*. (Letter to the editor.) *Lancet* 1988; 1: 1398.

190 Scandinavian Simvastatin Survival Study Group. Randomised trial of cholesterol lowering in 4444 patients with coronary heart disease: the Scandinavian Simvastatin Survival Study (4S). *Lancet* 1994; 344: 1383–9.

191 Naylor CD, Chen E, Strauss B. Method enthusiasm: does the method of reporting trial results alter perceptions of therapeutic effectiveness? *Ann Intern Med* 1992; 117: 916–21.

192 In ref. 14, p. 42.

* 193 Peto R, Pike MC, Armitage P *et al*. Design and analysis of randomized trials requiring prolonged observation of each patient. I Introduction and design. *Br J Cancer* 1977; 34: 585–612.

* 194 Peto R, Pike MC, Armitage P *et al*. Design and analysis of randomized trials requiring prolonged observation of each patient. II Analysis and examples. *Br J Cancer* 1978; 35: 1–39.

195 Machin D, Gardner MJ. Calculating confidence intervals for survival time analyses. *BMJ* 1988; 296: 1369–71.

Index

Index

Index